# RADICAL
# LOVE

# Zachary Levi

# RADICAL
# LOVE

*Learning to Accept
Yourself and Others*

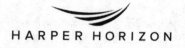

HARPER HORIZON

*I dedicate this book to my mom, Susy,*
*and all those like her, who left us before knowing*
*how truly loved they really were.*

# CONTENTS

In telling my story, my deepest desire is
to encourage you to tell your own.


Then, perhaps, we can finally learn to radically
love, radically accept, and radically forgive
ourselves and each other, at last.

# The Book in Your Hand

The book you have in your hand was supposed to have been in your hand a year ago. It was written. All but finished. Just a few final tweaks and I was ready to hit *send*. It was, I hoped, a powerful and compelling tale of my mental health journey from the depths of despair and depression to recovery, culminating in my greatest—or, at the very least, best-known—professional achievement: being cast in the title role of the movie *Shazam!*

At that point, the subtitle of the book was going to be "From Suicide to Superhero." Because that was my story. I had reached the point where I didn't want to go on living, and then a month later I was back to work with a new lease on life. I'd been to hell and back and come through, more or less, in one piece. I wasn't magically "cured"; I still had issues to work on and I was working on them. But I had an uplifting tale to tell about hope, perseverance, acceptance, and, above all, radical love. Wanting to share my experience to help others, I started doing interviews with various podcasts and publications, and a very kind editor at HarperCollins reached out to inquire if I'd be interested in putting my thoughts and experiences down in a book.

I'd never once imagined my life story being important enough to take up a whole book that other human beings would pay actual money for. Still, given how vital and important it is for our society to address the subject of mental health, I felt that if I could use my story and whatever platform I've been given to help anyone out there who's struggling, it would be a worthwhile thing to do. I think vulnerability is important. I think it's a superpower. It feels awkward and scary to be open and real with people, but it has only ever brought positive things into my life. Plus, I genuinely feel it's a part of my responsibility to talk about the struggles I've had. *Maybe I can write something informative and illuminating*, I thought, *and hopefully even a little entertaining as well.* So I sat down and poured my heart out and wrote the book. It was pretty much ready to go and the sequel to *Shazam!* was just about ready to film, and then: Boom.

The whole world shut down.

Then it exploded.

In the spring and summer of 2020, the Covid-19 pandemic hit and sociopolitical unrest exploded nationwide in the wake of the killing of George Floyd. My work and my life ground to a halt, and my mental health cratered along with them. The relative stability and peace of mind I'd fought so hard to build proved to be far more fragile than I'd allowed myself to believe.

The manuscript for this book sat and sat on my desk, waiting for my final edits. I was so crippled by anxiety and depression I couldn't even bring myself to look at it. And besides, did anyone out there want to read "From Suicide to Superhero and Back to Suicide Again"? I didn't imagine they would. I picked up the phone, called my editor, and explained where I was and how I didn't think I could make my deadline.

"But that's not even the biggest problem," I said.

"What is it?" he asked.

"The ending," I replied. "It doesn't work anymore. Because I didn't come through it, and I'm definitely not okay."

So the book went on hold along with the rest of my life, a rough year went by, and now here I am back at the keyboard, typing again. Not merely because I'm in a better place, though I feel that I am, but because that rough year brought me to a place where I finally understood the ending. I came to the very, very, very hard

realization that my mental health journey doesn't *have* an ending.
I'm not "fixed." I may never be "fixed." But it's okay that I'm not.
I may never be able to repair all of my brokenness, but I can love
myself in spite of my brokenness. I understand that now. So even
though my journey hasn't come to an end, I have come to the end
of the story I want to share with you.

Which leaves us only one question: Where to begin?

Honestly, we could pick any number of points. We could start
with me throwing myself onto a community theater stage to get
the love and approval of strangers that I never got at home. We
could start with my Grandma Pat chasing my naked mom out of
the house with a butcher knife. Given what we know about how
generational trauma works, we could start in Civil War–era
Missouri with my maternal great-great-great grandfather's drinking problem. Or maybe try my dad's side in Colonial New England
and start with my great-great-great-great-great-great-great-great-
great-great grandmother being put on trial for witchcraft. That
could be fun. But I don't know that we need to go back that far.
This story, the one I want to tell here, starts out the same way a lot
of stories do nowadays.

It starts with a ping.

# *The Way Things Work*

My phone let out a *ping!* I reached into my pocket, pulled my phone out, and clicked on the notification to see an email from my agents back in Los Angeles. It was about an audition for the lead role in the new DC superhero movie, *Shazam!*

It looked interesting, but I immediately saw a problem. I knew the Shazam character a bit. As a kid, I'd always been more of a Marvel comic book fan than a DC comic book fan, but even among DC fans, Shazam—or Captain Marvel, as he was originally known— is a bit of a niche character. He's Billy Batson, the fifteen-year-old kid who only has to say a magic word, "Shazam!," and he's instantly transformed into a superhero, which is pretty much every kid's dream. I also knew that Shazam has an archnemesis, Black Adam, who's basically Shazam's Bizarro-World twin. The role of Black Adam had already been cast, and he was going to be played by Dwayne "The Rock" Johnson, former WWE world champion and current Biggest Action Movie Star in the World. Obviously, it was not lost on me that The Rock and I do not look like twins. It seemed to me like they were probably looking for a John Cena type of guy.

I read over the email a couple of times, thought about it for a bit, then emailed back. "Aren't they looking for dudes that are, at the very least, super jacked, if not super famous, for this?" I asked. And God bless the assistant, whose reply might as well have been: ¯\_(ツ)_/¯

It felt like my agency was throwing me a bone, trying to make me feel like I was in the mix for big projects while knowing full well that I had no shot at getting the job, so I declined, saying I didn't want to waste everyone's time. And that was that for me and Shazam: Wasn't meant to be. Was never going to happen. On to the next thing.

Or maybe there wouldn't be a next thing. I can say now that this was my real fear. It had been five years since my TV show *Chuck* had been canceled by NBC. I'd worked steadily since, but my phone wasn't ringing off the hook with major offers. I was secretly afraid that my run as an actor was all but finished. On top of that, while most of my friends were off getting hitched and settling down, my marriage had imploded, just like every other relationship I'd ever had. I was closing in on thirty-seven, alone, with no family. I'd packed my entire life into a U-Haul and moved to Austin from Los Angeles with big dreams that were going to change my life, dreams that had given me a newfound sense of mission and purpose, but now I was beginning to question whether I'd made a terrible mistake.

What I can say, in hindsight, is that I was suffering from a tremendous amount of anxiety at the time. I had, in fact, been wrestling with anxiety and depression and fear and self-loathing my entire life. I just hadn't known it. I knew that I got sad and that I had my ups and downs, but I 100 percent did not think of myself as someone with serious mental health issues. I didn't know what anxiety and depression really were, at least not from a clinical point of view. When I finally did learn the depths of their meaning, it was a revelation: "Wait a minute . . . if this is what anxiety is, then this is what I've been feeling almost every waking moment for most of my life."

Up until that summer I'd always managed to white-knuckle my way through my problems, self-medicating and finding ways to keep myself propped up without ever realizing how emotionally fragile I was. And when it came to the subject of my own mental health, I was functionally illiterate.

Coming to terms with the full scope of my ignorance about mental health was upsetting for me. I'm a person who's always prided myself on my ability to tackle complex problems and figure them out. One of my favorite books as kid was this oversized picture book called *The Way Things Work*. It had page after page of these fun cross-section illustrations showing you "This is how a pulley works" and "This is how an elevator works." I used to sit and look through it for hours. I've always been fascinated with that kind of stuff. Even though I'm an actor, and therefore an artist by trade, I think I've always had more of an engineer's brain. That brain has helped me many times in my career, having the ability to analyze how the business of Hollywood operates, taking the system apart to figure out the best way to navigate it. But that same mind was completely flummoxed when it came to understanding how its own inner mechanisms functioned. I didn't understand the cause and effect between the traumas I'd experienced as a child and the behaviors I was wrestling with as an adult. I didn't understand that so much of my insecurity came from outsourcing my sense of self-worth to forces beyond my control, such as whether or not Hollywood casting directors liked me. I didn't understand that the reason my marriage had ended wasn't because I'd failed, but because I was broken.

When you don't understand how a machine works you can't ever hope to repair it, and because our understanding of mental illness is so poor, the ways we try to cope with it often end up making it worse. We don't respond to our negative feelings—we react to them. To respond to something is to carefully weigh the causes and consequences of a decision while understanding our own motivations for making that decision. To react is to let our reptile brains operate by knee-jerk reflex, leading us into cycles and patterns of self-destructive behavior. We explode with road rage when we're stuck in traffic. We lock ourselves in our rooms and block out everything except that inner voice telling us that we're worthless and stupid. We turn to drugs and alcohol to try to numb ourselves. We even do things that don't seem to make a whole lot of sense, like turning down once-in-a-lifetime opportunities to star in major Hollywood superhero movies.

When I passed on the audition for *Shazam!*, I told everyone, including myself, that it would be a waste of everyone's time because of the Dwayne Johnson thing. The truth is it was mostly a knee-jerk reflex of self-sabotage. I had been through so many career disappointments, and my initial enthusiasm for moving to Austin was being battered by waves of panic and self-doubt. With my confidence at such a low ebb, I couldn't bear the thought of being rejected again. If I'd gone back to LA and tried out for that job and failed to get it, it would have been part of my destruction. So my subconscious lapsed into that old, familiar defense mechanism: let me reject them before they have a chance to reject me. And that's how I let such a golden opportunity slip away.

But, like I said, I didn't know any of that at the time. In my mind, I had arrived in Texas for a bold, new adventure that was going to lift me up and fill my life with the meaning and purpose it had been lacking. In reality, I was standing on the edge of a cliff, and the ground beneath my feet was about to give way.

# RADICAL
## LOVE

# ONE

# Stop Running

Taking care of your mind should be no more embarrassing than taking care of your teeth. We all need to be proactive—to brush and floss, our minds to root out the lies we tell ourselves and the bad programming that drives so much of our behavior. We don't. We do the opposite. We pretend and project out to the world that "I'm great!" and "We're great!" and "Everything's fine!" But it's not always fine, and because we refuse to admit that, we do nothing, and all of a sudden what started out as a little cavity is now in need of a root canal.

. . .

Society places a terrible stigma on mental illness. We judge people for it in ways that we never would for other kinds of health issues. If you tell someone you're physically ill, they say, "Oh gosh. I'm so sorry. What's the matter? Talk to me." There's no stigma attached to it. From cancer to the common cold, people want to make sure you're okay. But when you swap out "physical illness" with "mental illness," then people seem to start pondering, *Well, how unstable is this person? Is it time for a straitjacket and a rubber room?* Which makes us ashamed to talk about it. We shouldn't be, but we are—and I was, like so many other people.

It took a long time for me to recognize how much help and healing I needed. When I moved to Texas, even though I didn't fully realize it yet, I felt hopeless and alone. I'd been white-knuckling through my problems for so long, barely holding it together, and I was petrified of what people would think of me if they knew the truth about what a broken, horrible person I was—or thought I was. My marriage had begun and ended disastrously. My mother had passed away, which I thought I'd dealt with but in fact had not. And my work, which had always been the load-bearing wall keeping my self-esteem propped up, had started to crumble.

Even when I was doing well, Hollywood had never been a healthy place for me. I don't know if it's a healthy place for anyone, really, and from the time I started booking jobs in television, even at the age of nineteen, it was unbelievable to me the way the system worked. Or, rather, didn't work. It was broken to the point of being not only inhumane, but also inefficient. Like too many industries, Hollywood is a place where the people in power will do whatever they can, within the law and sometimes not within the law, to make as much money as they can for themselves, and because of that, it's a place where human life isn't valued. Not more than money, anyway. For actors, it can be emotionally debilitating. For crew members—everyday people trying to earn a decent wage—it can be downright exploitive.

Trauma bends our minds into incorrect thinking patterns, so much so that we can barely see or think our way around them.

Within a few months of being inside the Hollywood machine, looking at it with my engineer's brain, I thought, *There has got to be a better way.* Moving to Austin was an attempt to find that better way. I wanted to build a new kind of studio, a better machine, a place where people who love film and who love to tell stories can live and work and play, and find the feelings of community and connection that don't exist in Hollywood anymore. After seventeen years of dreaming about it, praying about it, and waiting for it, that summer I finally decided to do it. Searching the country for the right location, I found Austin, which felt like the Promised Land. It was groovy. It had an incredible artistic vibe—and no personal state income tax. I came out with a couple of buddies, and we drove all around and started scouting parcels of land around the city. "This is it," I decided. "I can feel it in my gut. I have to do this." So I sold my house in Los Angeles, put most of my belongings in storage, packed everything I would need to start my new life into a U-Haul, hitched it to the back of my Ford Raptor, and headed east. I rented a small house in the neighborhood of Travis Heights to serve as a temporary home base while I closed on a gorgeous parcel of land I'd found—seventy-five acres on the Colorado River—with the hope of finding investors to come on board and help make my dream a reality.

Most of my friends didn't understand what I was doing. I'm sure they thought I was making a huge mistake. They were probably right. It wasn't the smartest idea, at least not in the impulsive way I'd done it. Once I arrived in Texas, the initial rush of adrenaline and enthusiasm that had carried me there started to wear off, a work project I'd been counting on fell through, and I started feeling waves of panic and doubt.

Still trying to keep up my personal and professional commitments, I boarded a flight for a weeklong trip to the Philippines in my role as an ambassador for Operation Smile, an organization that provides life-changing surgeries to children born with cleft palates, primarily in poor and developing countries. I was taking a camera crew and tagging along with a medical mission to make a short film highlighting the group's work. That was tough. I'm an empathetic person by nature. I see people cry and I immediately start to well up. I see people in pain and can't help but feel their pain. And that's me on a good day. On a bad day, it's a real problem. Even the slightest reminder that pain exists in the world can send me over the edge. So, at a time when I was already in a fragile emotional state, it was probably not the best idea to surround myself with third-world poverty and suffering. But being unaware of how fragile my emotional state was, that's what I did.

The hardest day for me was when we left the hospital and went out to the surrounding farms. We visited this family, a single mother raising three children, one of whom had a cleft lip and palate. They were living in a makeshift shanty, a shack with stick walls and a thatched roof and a dirt floor, and this woman, the mother, took so much pride in her shack. You can't clean dirt. It's dirt. Still, she had a broom and she was sweeping the dirt floors, brushing away the little rocks and sticks to make it smooth, to make the best home she could for her family. This family had nothing, and at the same time they had everything. They had a mother loving them, taking care of them. She'd been waiting three years for the boy to get surgery. They lived ninety minutes from the nearest hospital, and she had to carry him on a half-hour walk to the nearest village to catch a buggy for an hour-long ride into the city for the screening.

To see a mother doing that for her child, acting out of pure, selfless love, was both life-affirming and heartbreaking, because it was something so alien to my own experience growing up. I started ruminating on all the horrible things going on in my own life, which then made me feel even more guilty. Because who was I to feel ungrateful? "Oh, woe is you, white American actor boy. You've got so much and you're sad? Who do you think you are?" I was tumbling into a spiral of self-loathing, eviscerating myself. My subconscious kept telling me all manner of horrible shit: *You're so stupid. You're a fucking idiot. You fucked everything up. You never should have come here.*

Very quickly, I found that I couldn't cope. I was overwhelmed by the sight of these kids, their families, and the debilitating medical problems they were struggling with. Once we started filming, I was stumbling around in a fog, incapable of making basic decisions about what shots or interviews we needed to line up. Luckily, I'd brought along my good friend Justin to serve as a producer and my brother-in-law, Ian, to work as our main camera operator. They stepped in to organize the crew. Meanwhile, I kept having to walk off and find a spot where I could be alone and cry. I normally don't have a problem with crying; I think it's a beautiful thing, not to mention therapeutic and cathartic. But you need to have a handle on that shit, and I did not.

I managed to hold myself together for the rest of the trip. On the last night of the mission, our hosts threw us a party and somebody came out with all the traditional Filipino delicacies, including *balut*, a local street food you can't get in America. It's like a hard-boiled duck egg, only the egg has been fertilized, so it's really a hard-boiled duck embryo. All the Westerners were whipping out their iPhones and taking videos, daring each other to try it, so I did. It was . . . interesting. It tasted like a salty scrambled egg, but the texture felt gelatinous and slightly crunchy all at the same time. I got a cool Instagram post out of it, and I'm fairly certain I got a stomach parasite out of it, too, because on the flight home my gut started tying itself in knots. Which, on top of the waves of anxiety and self-loathing I was already experiencing, was the last thing I needed.

> Crying is critical to the healing process. It helps us release pain and trauma, which can help lead to acceptance and peace.

By the time I got back, it felt like everything in my life was coming apart at the same time. I couldn't have scripted it to be any worse. It was a perfect storm, literally. Hurricane Harvey hit the Texas coast that week. Houston got the worst of it, but even up in Austin it was dark and cloudy and pouring rain for days. I couldn't leave the house. I was infected with this parasite, totally constipated, nothing coming out; I could hear the gurgling and bubbling in my intestines as this thing was eating away at my insides. I had crazy insomnia from the jet lag. I was up all night, looking around this empty house, looking at everything I'd brought packed up in boxes, berating myself for making such a horrible mistake with my life by coming out here. *Look what you've done, Zac. You stupid piece of shit. You've failed at everything. You had it, and you fucked it all up.*

The decision to move to Texas had filled me with excitement. I was so certain that coming out here would give me renewed purpose. I was sacrificing my own money, my own time, my own resources to give people in my industry a better life and more community and better pay—to help build a better world. I'd been so gung ho about the move that I'd even quit smoking and drinking. It was going to be a new day, a clean break. And it was. But it was too clean. I was living in a new place where I knew no one. I was completely removed from my work, my friends, my family. I had no one to support me, nothing to distract me. I didn't even have a pack of American Spirits or a bottle of Jameson to reach for to help me self-medicate my way through as I always had.

You can't run away from yourself, so there's no point in trying. Yet in my stubbornness and denial and fear, it's what I had been doing for years. Here's how stupid I was: before leaving for Austin, I'd even broken up with my girlfriend, *and she was from Austin*. She's a beautiful and wonderful person and her family lives there and she wanted to stay with me, but I threw it all away because of all the same insecurities and self-doubts that have ruined every other relationship I'd ever been in up to that point. Unbeknownst to me, all the things I'd given up and left behind were the very things that had been keeping me afloat. And maybe I could have held on if I'd only lost some of those things, but I also lost the most important thing. I lost God.

Back in LA, planning the move to Texas, I felt that God was present in my life. I felt His hand guiding me every step of the way, and I was so certain I was doing the right thing. Now, here I was. I'd come to the Promised Land and I'd done what He wanted me to do, and it all felt like a terrible mistake. I felt totally abandoned by God. For the first time in my life, I didn't know if I believed in God, or if there even was a God. For the first time in my life, I was completely and utterly alone with nobody and nothing but myself.

And that's when the bottom fell out.

# Get Help

If you're feeling overwhelmed, run-down, fearful, stressed out, anxious, depressed, alone, or anything that may be robbing you of your peace or your joy, talk to someone. Do *not* believe the lie that you are going through this alone. Because you aren't. You could be sitting next to someone, right this second, who struggles with the same issues that you do. Maybe that person can help you. We are all in this together.

· · ·

From the minute we come into this world, even though we're not aware of it, we're trying to feel that we belong, that we matter. We look to our parents and our friends and our family and our school and our society, and we ask them, "Who am I? Do I have worth in this world? Do I have purpose in this life?"

The answer, without question, is "*Yes. You do.*" Unfortunately, most of the time we don't hear that answer. Unfortunately, too many of us have parents who don't make us feel as if we belong. Unfortunately, we belong to a society that prioritizes all the wrong things—things like money and fame and attractiveness and over-all status—forcing us to judge ourselves against all the wrong standards, standards by which we always come up short. So then we find ourselves alone in the darkness, where the voices come for us and tell us how stupid and ugly and worthless we are. But it's a lie. It's a fuckin' lie. You belong here simply because you *are* here.

God created every single one of us with our own inherent worth
and value and dignity. Mental illness is the lie that undermines
that truth.

In fact, not only is it a lie, it's a lie that begets more lies in turn,
as lies often do. One of the most insidious of those lies is that your
problems are yours alone. Because you've never been inside someone else's head to feel the pain they feel, you're convinced that
you're the only person suffering like this—that you're the only
person who has *ever* suffered like this. Which is why you can be
surrounded by friends and family telling you "It's okay" and still
feel so horribly alone. It's also why the situation feels so hopeless.
Why even ask for help when nobody could possibly help you?
Because if you're the only one with this problem, what are the
chances of doctors ever diagnosing and treating you? You're so
broken that no one will ever be able to find the cure. Of course,
none of that is true. There are millions of people who hurt the
same way that you hurt. There are thousands of doctors and therapists who understand how to treat you and how to help you. But
you can't see that because the thing that you're sick with comes
with an absence of hope, an absence of faith—the inability to see
yourself and life clearly.

The week of Hurricane Harvey I plunged into a despair and a
darkness deeper than anything else I'd ever experienced. I was
paralyzed, physically and emotionally. I could barely sleep at all,
and when I was awake, it was to sit or lie catatonic on the couch.
And every sleepless night I was alone in my room, on my knees,
crying, weeping, sobbing, yelling out to a God who wasn't there.
"Why?! Why?! Why?! What have I *done*? I am *lost*! I need you. I need
your *help*! I need it *now*!"

Outside in the world, August gave way to September and people
were out living their lives, but inside my house time had collapsed.
The days and weeks blurred together. I had a massive to-do list I
needed to tackle, suitcases to unpack, boxes to move out of storage, and I couldn't do any of it. When in states of major turmoil,

I fall into this place where the minutiae of life will bury me. I'll have a hard time making decisions, even about the smallest things. I think there are two broad categories of anxious people: those who are anxious about things that they can't control, and those who are anxious about the things they can. With major events outside my control, such as getting hit by a truck on the freeway, I've always had a much easier time being like, "Well, okay, it is what it is." I've always been far more anxious about what I *can* control. I get stuck trying to figure out the perfect way to do the thing and I think, *Don't fuck this up. Don't fuck this up. Don't fuck this up.* The thing *has* to be perfect, because if a thing is not perfect, it's a failure, and failures don't receive love. And why do I think this way? Because that's the way I was programmed as a kid by my parents.

I can remember standing in the kitchen of my Austin rental, staring at this box of plates, not knowing which cabinet I should put them in, thinking whichever cabinet I picked was going to be the wrong one and then the whole kitchen would be ruined forever—this kitchen that I was only going to be using for two months, tops. My self-talk, as always, was horrible. *Why did I even buy these stupid plates in the first place when I know I'm a worthless piece of shit who doesn't even know what to do with them?* So I gave up. I left the plates in the box, left the cabinets empty.

I didn't want to reach out to anyone. I felt so worthless I didn't think anyone would care—I didn't think anyone *should* care. Luckily, I have better friends than that. People were calling and texting to check in, realizing that I was not okay. I had several friends get on a plane and fly in to look after me: my friend Justin, my friends Hillary and Sarah. They flew in, helped me clean, made me food, and did all the other basic tasks that I was no longer capable of doing.

Then they'd sit and talk with me. "It's okay," they'd say. "It's okay." And I'd be crying, over and over again, "It's *not* okay! *Nothing* is okay." Everything felt meaningless. I couldn't see any purpose to my life. Because if there is no God, if we are just sacks of meat, shuffling around, filling our days with some random purpose of our own making until we all kind of peter out around age eighty-five, then what's the fucking point?

I didn't want to be alive anymore. I wasn't thinking about killing myself, not the way I had three years before when my marriage ended, which was the last time I'd felt anything close to this kind of darkness. That time I'd stood on the balcony of my hotel, looking down, wondering if the fall from thirteen stories would be enough to kill me. That time I'd put the knife to my wrist, trying to remember if you're supposed to go crossways or longways, which one does the job and which one slices the tendons and fucks up your arm. That time I came close, but I couldn't allow myself to think that way now. Now, there was someone else I had to think about.

People say that suicide is the most selfish thing you can do because it's inflicting pain on the people who care about you. But when you're in the depths of despair, it certainly doesn't feel that way; it feels like you're such a burden on everyone that by killing yourself you're doing the world a favor. But even in the depths of my pain, I was self-aware enough to think about my nephew, Gryffin. My younger sister, Shekinah, had given birth to Gryffin about eighteen months earlier. She and I are close, and I knew if I killed myself, it would destroy her, which in turn would leave this boy growing up without the healthy mom he deserved, and I couldn't bring myself do that to him. Trauma and abuse had haunted our family for generations, passed down from my grandmother to my mother to me and my sisters. I knew that I couldn't be the one to pass that on again. That thought was the only thing that kept me out of a coffin.

Since I couldn't bring myself to commit suicide, I was left with simply wishing that I could go to sleep and not wake up. Every night I'd put my head down and hope that some kind of natural cause would take me in the night. Then nobody could blame me for it. Nobody could say I was being selfish. It would just be one of those tragic things, you know? But that relief never came. Every morning I'd wake up and I'd still be there, still my same pathetic, worthless self.

Days passed, a week maybe. One afternoon I woke up and realized there was no food in the house. If I was going to eat, like it or not, I would have to go outside and be in the world. I got dressed and went out to my truck and drove off in search of sustenance. About five minutes up the road, I saw a sign for Chi'Lantro. I'd never been, but it was food and it was there and I didn't particularly care about anything in the moment, including what I ate, so I stopped.

The darkness is lying to you. Your trauma is lying to you. You matter in this world. You add value to this world. You are wonderfully made.

Chi'Lantro, as its hybrid name suggests, is a fast-casual, Korean-Mexican fusion restaurant. I pulled into the parking lot, found a spot, and as I braced myself to get out and go inside, all of a sudden I got hit with a severe panic attack. I was clutching the steering wheel and slamming my back against the seat, crying and yelling like I'd done at home, screaming out to God, "What the *fuck* is going on?! I am *lost*! I am *done*! Give me a *sign*. Give me *something*, because I don't know what's happening to me and I don't want to live anymore!" That went on for I don't know how long. Five, ten minutes maybe. Finally, I pulled myself together, took a deep breath, did my best to wipe the tears away from my red, puffy eyes, got out of the truck, and went inside.

The place was completely empty, save for me, the guy at the cash register, and a couple of people cooking in the back. I walked up to the counter and stared up at the menu. It was one of those build-your-own-bowl situations, which nearly broke me. Talk about analysis paralysis. I kept stumbling and stammering and doubling back and changing my mind about what I wanted. Everything I did felt wrong, which the nasty voice in my head was more than happy to point out for me. *Way to go,* idiot. *Can't even do this right. Can't even order fucking food for yourself. You're gonna fuck this up the same way you always fuck everything up.*

Finally, I managed to get my order out, the guy rang me up, and I walked over to a table to sit down, alone. A few minutes later, the same guy came over with my tray and set it down in front of me. I looked up with my puffy, bloodshot eyes and managed a quick nod, expecting him to turn and leave. He didn't. There was an awkward pause.

"Um . . . sir?" he said. "Are you okay? Can . . . can we help you?"

When your Chi'Lantro server is asking you if you need help, that's when you know you're in trouble.

I thanked him and politely declined. I genuinely was grateful that this complete stranger was showing me such generosity in the moment, but it was a telling sign. All my life, no matter what was going on with me, no matter how depressed or anxious I felt on the inside, I always managed to put on a cheerful, positive act for the world. But now I'd reached the point where I couldn't even do that; I couldn't even put on a happy face long enough to make it through lunch.

> When you start to be critical of yourself, see it as the lie that it is. Take a deep breath in, then let the lie go as you breathe out.

The minute I was back in my truck, I started weeping again, muttering to myself, "What am I doing? What's going on?" It was like when you see homeless people talking to themselves, because who else are they going to talk to? Nobody talks to them anymore. And that's when you really start to feel like you're losing your mind: when you have to talk to yourself in order to not be completely alone. I felt like I didn't even know what was real. I didn't think the walls were melting or anything like that, but I couldn't make sense of this world and who I was and how I fit into it. Nothing made sense. All I knew was that whatever was going on with me was a real five-alarm fire. I needed help, and I didn't know how to ask for it.

One of the friends who'd come out to visit me, my buddy Justin, had been worried enough that he'd taken it upon himself to google the local treatment options, and he discovered that the Dell Seton Medical Center at the University of Texas has a psychiatric wing where you can admit yourself on an emergency basis. Justin had also told me what everyone with mental health issues needs to hear. "Don't be ashamed to go," he said. "If you need to go, and there's a place to go, *go*."

## THERAPY

Having come through to the other side of intensive therapy, I now know how important and necessary therapy is. We get so wrapped up in our own narratives, the stories we tell ourselves about ourselves, that we can't see any truth other than the twisted one we've constructed to justify what we do. Those narratives might be debilitating because they're unfairly negative, like when we tell ourselves that we're stupid or worthless or unworthy of love. Or they might be debilitating because they're positive to the point of being delusional or narcissistic, like believing that we're always right about everything because we're smarter than everyone else. Whatever our individual issues are, we all have bad programming that day by day is crippling us, but even as it's crippling us it's also comforting us through its familiarity. We retreat to it and take refuge in it. We avoid anything that challenges it, because it's the only defense mechanism we know.

So we avoid therapists. We avoid them precisely because they're going to do what we're scared to do: dismantle the defense mechanisms we've come to rely on. Because a therapist is, or should be, an objective third party with no investment in maintaining the lies and stories we prop ourselves up with. And when we share our stories with a therapist, it's like exposing them to sunlight or holding them up to a mirror. We can start to see our bad programming for what it is, and the lies that we tell ourselves about ourselves will, hopefully, begin to crumble and turn to dust.

Opening up to friends and family doesn't accomplish the same goal. Friends and family are a wonderful, necessary place to start. We absolutely should open up to them and admit we need help. But our friends and family are not objective, disinterested third parties. They have their own agendas, misperceptions, and biases. People in my life have never known how to counsel me. To start with, my friends didn't live my childhood, so how could they possibly understand the trauma I've gone through? Second, I had always been a stubborn person who didn't think I had that many problems to begin with. And finally, on most days, regardless of what was going on inside me, I projected the image of someone who's chipper and upbeat.

That situation was further complicated by the fact that so many of my friends and family members worked for me and were dependent on me financially. I had massive trust issues because of that. I could never be sure if the advice they were giving me was in my best interest, or theirs.

Merely talking to God doesn't cut it either. Prayer is a wonderful thing, and it has given me solace on countless occasions, but it is not a substitute for therapy. If your head's not right, and if you don't see reality the way that reality actually is, then prayer alone isn't going to help you see it. Prayer offers a time to reflect, to look inward, to be present with God. But prayer doesn't hold up a cold, unflinching mirror to your life the way therapy does. Therapy breaks down our defenses and exposes us so that we can finally begin to understand ourselves and build ourselves back up. No matter how healthy we think we are, we all need it.

Even as miserable and suicidal as I'd been, the idea of seeking institutional help was possibly even more terrifying. It was something that could greatly affect my livelihood. If I walked into a psychiatric hospital and someone recognized me and said, "Hey, there's that guy from TV," my career could seriously be in jeopardy. I could see the headlines on *TMZ*: "Star of NBC's *Chuck* Admitted to Hospital over Nervous Breakdown." But in that moment, I was so messed up and so terrified of what I might do to myself, I decided I didn't have any choice. *I have to go*, I thought. *I have to take the risk and do this.* And besides, I was already convinced I'd screwed up my entire life. Even if I fully exposed myself to the world as a crazy person, how could that possibly make my situation any worse? So I went.

I pulled out of the Chi'Lantro parking lot and drove straight across town to the medical center. The whole way over I was beating myself up about it, my terrible self-talk turned up to eleven. *Am I really doing this? Am I doing the right thing? Yes, you idiot. What the hell else are you going to do? What are your options?* I arrived at the hospital, parked, went inside, and found my way to the psychiatric wing. The nurse at the desk took one look at me, saw the same red, puffy face that had concerned the Chi'Lantro guy, and realized right away that there was a problem. She processed me and told me to have a seat. "Wait here," she said, "and a doctor will be with you shortly."

Looking around, I quickly realized this was no regular waiting room. I was in a special waiting room, for special people, like me. Most of the patients all looked zonked out on different heavy medications, most of them slouched down in their vinyl chairs, eyes glued to a television up on the wall. I remember there was some sort of horribly violent action movie on, people mowing each other down with machine guns. Even in my messed-up state, I was keenly aware of the dark irony of playing this kind of film for people wrestling with anxiety, depression, or thoughts of self-harm.

Finally, I was called in to meet with someone, not a therapist or a doctor, but a social worker. She started going through this standard form, asking me all these generic, open-ended questions, such as "How are you feeling?" and "Why are you feeling this way?" Inside, all I wanted to do was scream, *"I don't know why I'm feeling this way! Otherwise, I wouldn't be here!"* Luckily, I was still in touch with reality enough to know that this social worker was a nice person who, God bless her, was just doing her job. I didn't scream, but I still didn't know how to answer anything she was asking me. I felt like I was on another planet of despondence and fear and anxiety, wrestling with deep and complex issues that I had no understanding of. I didn't have the words to explain anything.

At the same time, I had so much bottled up inside me that I was also like, "Where do you want me to start?" So I basically rambled, from my mother's emotional abuse to her drinking problem to my absent father to the suicidal thoughts I had on my honeymoon. Then there was the fact that I couldn't leave my house, that I'd lost faith in God, that I was crying in my car. And on and on and on. None of it made any sense. I felt terrible for this poor lady who was surely staring down at her form, clueless as to what box she should check for the human disaster sitting across from her.

Eventually, a doctor arrived. After taking a moment to look over my intake forms and ask me a few questions, she presented me with my options. Option number one was that they could give me a mild sedative and send me home. Option number two was to check myself in for a twenty-four-hour watch while the doctors determined how to proceed. Option number one seemed like a joke. This sedative they offered me was something you can get over the counter. It's the equivalent of taking a Benadryl. I couldn't believe it. All I could think was, *Are you* shitting *me? That's it? I am* dying, *and that's the best you can give me?*

On the one hand, I understand why hospitals can't give out powerful psychoactive medications to people when they haven't even determined a diagnosis. But on the other hand, if I showed up at the emergency room with a broken leg, I feel certain they'd give me something way stronger than a fucking Benadryl, and whatever was happening to my mind was worse than a broken leg. Therein lies the riddle of mental health. Even a severe and obvious symptom, like a grown man crying and wailing at the ceiling, doesn't point to a specific cause or a clear-cut course of treatment. It's often the case that nobody, not even the doctor, knows what to do at first.

Which left me with option number two: checking myself in. The minute she raised the possibility, I balked. When you're an actor, anytime you star in a movie or a TV show, the studio takes out an insurance policy on you. For the duration of the production, your health and well-being are very much their business. Over the course of my career, and even in my personal life, I've filled out hundreds of forms and contracts, and a lot of them ask, "Have you ever been hospitalized for a mental health condition?" All of a sudden, I wasn't just panicked about the public finding out that I was in this place, I was paranoid in a "this will go down on your permanent record" kind of way.

I gave the doctor a long look and took a deep breath. Then I said, "Okay. I think I'm going to take the sedative and go home. Thank you very much."

And in that moment I felt, not better, but a sense of calm, almost relief. My feelings of anxiety and panic momentarily subsided. Because if these truly were my only two options—taking a Benadryl or being institutionalized—then I really was doomed. And if I was doomed, then there was nothing left for me to worry about. I got up from my chair, almost like a zombie, and shuffled back out to my truck.

That night I called my sister Shekinah, which I'd been reluctant to do. Shekinah's not only my sister, she's also one of my best friends and closest confidantes. She'd worked for me as my personal assistant for years; I relied on her for a lot. She had also been one of the biggest opponents of my moving to Texas, and I was scared to admit to her how much I was struggling. But after I explained what was going on, she said, "Maybe you should go away, to a facility."

"Maybe so," I replied.

"What about Promises?" she said, referring to the drug-and-alcohol rehab in Malibu where Hollywood's rich and famous go to dry out.

"Promises?" I said. "I'm not an addict, Shekinah. My problem is that I'm broken and I need healing. I'm open to going somewhere, but it's got to be the right place, and it's got to be a place of deep healing."

"Okay," she said. "Don't worry. I'm on it."

My sister is one of those people who, when given a mission, does not stop until it's done. She'll exhaust every option, leave no stone unturned, checking and double-checking every detail. And that night, tasked with saving her brother's life, she went online and started digging through every corner of the internet to find the right facility for me. By the time I woke up the next morning, she was already emailing me ideas. Eventually, she forwarded me some info on a group in Connecticut that was created for corporate CEOs and the like. She vetted it thoroughly, even calling and talking to the owner. Then she called me to discuss it.

"Zac," she said, "I think this is the place. It's great."

I looked it up online and browsed the website while we spoke. It wasn't cheap. None of the good options are, which is yet another hurdle keeping people from getting the treatment they need. Ultimately, after going back and forth about it, I decided to pull the trigger. I was blessed and fortunate enough to have the money, which not many people do, and what good would it do to save the money if at the end of the day I was dead? Having any amount of money in the bank doesn't mean a whole lot if you can't bring yourself to get up off the living room floor.

Shekinah called the organization, booked my stay, and started making the travel arrangements. For the next few weeks, I did my best to hold myself together. I started seeing a local psychiatrist. He couldn't do much for me in the short period of time I had before leaving, but he did prescribe me some medication, a combination of carbamazepine and Lexapro. I don't know if it helped, and I'd always been extremely resistant to the idea of being on medication, but at that point I was willing to try anything.

At the same time, I went about wrapping up loose ends so I could get away for a month, which included a quick trip out to LA to do some housekeeping with my agents and managers. When we sat down, I told them that for the next month I'd be off the grid. "At a healing retreat," I told them, which they understood and were fully supportive of. I didn't share the specifics about what the place was or how bad things had gotten for me, but then I didn't need to; it was obvious to everyone that I was in rough shape. We talked a bit about possible jobs and business that might come up while I was out, and it was then that I learned that the role of Shazam had basically been cast. "They found their guy," my agent said, "and it's a guy who's similar to you. You could have had a real shot at that." It was disappointing to hear, but not getting cast as a superhero was hardly my most pressing concern in the moment; I was far more preoccupied with remaining alive.

I flew back to Texas and the morning of September 29, my thirty-seventh birthday, the papers came through for me to close on my land outside Austin. I drove down to the real estate title office and pulled into the parking lot in a total state of panic about the whole thing. Was I about to make the biggest mistake of my life? Was I a complete idiot? Just as I had outside Chi'Lantro, I sat there clutching the steering wheel, rocking back and forth and crying and screaming for a good ten minutes. Then I wiped away the tears, went inside, and put on a big, happy show for everybody, being that guy from TV, the jokey extrovert's extrovert. I signed the papers, shook everyone's hand, went back to my truck, and broke down weeping uncontrollably again.

That night, some family and friends who'd flown into town took me out to dinner, doing their best to prop me up and keep me in decent spirits. I spent the next two days packing and getting ready, and on October 2, I took a car to the airport and boarded a plane for Connecticut.

I landed in the evening. It was already dark and a bit rainy out. A car was there to pick me up. It was about an hour-and-a-half drive to the place. I spent some of it chatting with the driver, doing my best to be affable and friendly. But most of the time I stared silently out the window. We arrived at the house, and I went through the check-in routine, filling out the necessary paperwork. Then I headed up to my room, closed the door behind me, and collapsed onto the bed.

For weeks, I'd been on my own in my house in Austin, feeling abandoned by everyone, including God. Even though I'd decided to commit to this program, I was deeply skeptical of it. I questioned that I would come out of it changed for the better. But I had already taken the most important step: I'd asked for help. I'd reached out from the darkness and my friends and family had grabbed my hand, which was enough to tell me I wasn't completely alone in this. As I eased my head back onto my pillow that night, I realized I was in a nice, warm house and there were people there who wanted to help me, good people who were there to console me and take care of me. I closed my eyes to sleep and, for the first time in months, allowed myself the tiniest bit of hope.

*Maybe it will be okay,* I thought. *Maybe I've got a chance.*

# THREE

# *Be Open*

Even though our knowledge of the human mind and body has increased a thousandfold over time, and miraculous breakthroughs of understanding do occur, many of the mysteries of existence remain beyond our grasp. We're constantly revising what we know about what we don't know. All throughout history, scientists have said, "We've got it! We've figured it out!" Then a few years go by, and it turns out everyone's assumptions were wrong. We grew up thinking that dinosaurs were these enormous reptiles. Then one day all the paleontologists said, "Well, it turns out they were more like enormous chickens." Nowhere is this truer than with mental health.

. . .

Mental illness is a subject that we don't talk about enough, that we don't understand enough, that we're scared to confront. In many cases, we're so ignorant we don't even know how much we don't know. My friends knew I was struggling, but they didn't fully grasp the depths of what I was struggling with. They wanted to help me and support me, but most of what I heard from them was "You seem unhappy." And I was unhappy, deeply unhappy. But none of them could put a finger on why, and neither could I. I'd been in and out of therapy a few times in my life, addressing symptoms here and there, doing little hit-and-runs—as they call them—on my various issues. But I'd never fully digested and metabolized what I needed to know in order to cope with all my pain and sadness and anger.

When I arrived in Connecticut, I didn't know what I didn't know. I didn't know what I was going to get out of it, and I didn't know who I was going to be on the other side of it. I was afraid I would turn into a version of myself that I didn't like. Part of me was afraid that because this wasn't a spiritual facility, I would come out of my experience with even less faith and less spirit than when I went in. I was so lost, all I knew for certain was that I wanted someone to tell me what the fuck was going on, to give me an answer, a capital-D diagnosis.

That is what many of us, wrongly, have come to expect from medicine and science. The truth, especially with mental health, is that there are still so many big questions to be answered—questions that get harder to address the more hubris we have in believing we understand them. We started out in a world where mental conditions like depression and schizophrenia were chalked up to sorcery and demons and witchcraft. Then it was Freud, and everything was about dreams and wanting to sleep with your mother. Then it was B. F. Skinner and behaviorism, where there's no free will and no human soul and we're all bodies with nerve endings driven by stimulus-response mechanisms that seek to maximize pleasure and avoid pain. For me, the most important and influential of these figures is Carl Jung, whom I consider the originator of the idea of radical acceptance—recognizing the darkness in yourself in order to understand the darkness in others. But the reality is that everyone is making their best guess. Nobody knows everything for sure. All of us should put our hands in the air and say, "We've been so fuckin' wrong about so many things, and all we want is to learn more to get closer to the truth." Ideally, we should want to know everything that affects us in every possible way. We should want to be the healthiest, strongest version of ourselves and go make the world a better place, and to do that, it's important to use the mental and spiritual and emotional exercises we need to dig into that stuff. Too often in life we pick a point on the horizon and say, "That's where I need to be, and all I need is the shortest route between here and there." But that's wrong. We have to accept that we don't always know where we're going and that we don't even know how to get there. We have to be open to the journey. We have to be open to discovery. We have to radically accept where we are in life right now.

My first morning in Connecticut, I was still struggling to do that. I woke up, got dressed, and walked downstairs, and a woman was there, sitting at a table and having a cup of coffee, waiting for me. She looked to be in her early fifties, petite and fair-skinned with shortish blonde hair. I sat down with her and we started chatting a bit, getting to know each other. Her name was Beth, and she was going to be my companion for the day. It was her job to escort me through all my various appointments.

This place I'd checked into worked like a kind of umbrella organization, bringing together different therapists, psychiatrists, doctors, and other mental health and wellness professionals. They all worked in their own private practices, but they coordinated together through this central agency to provide a holistic course of treatment.

When my sister and I first looked at the whole range of services and treatments they offered, I told the administrator I wanted all of them. "Throw the kitchen sink at me," I said. "'Let's pull out all the stops. Let's leave no stone unturned." What I ended up paying for was three weeks of intensive therapy, plus a fourth week of final, circle-up appointments with all the therapists where they'd give me their assessments, assign me homework, and send me on my way. The specialists I was scheduled to see included a psychiatrist, a psychotherapist, a dialectical behavioral therapist, a meditation therapist, an art therapist, a life coach, a nutritionist, and a trainer at the gym four days a week, plus Pilates and yoga twice a week.

Like I said, the kitchen sink.

For my appointments I'd get driven to the different therapists' offices in the surrounding area, scattered across quaint, picturesque New England towns. As a setting, Connecticut in October was stunning. The trees were in their full autumn blaze of red and orange and yellow. The house I stayed in was a cozy New England clapboard kind of place. It was right on Long Island Sound, and I could walk down a path to go and sit and hang out on the water and enjoy the crisp, fall air. There was a cook who'd come in to make lunch and dinner, and the companion assigned to you for the day would make your breakfast, do your laundry, take you to your appointments, and then drop you off at the end of the day back at the house. There were a number of different companions, and they would cycle through, assigned to different residents on different days. Like Beth, they were all middle-aged women, mostly wives and mothers who were semiretired. They were kind of like house moms, if you will.

As Beth and I sat chatting that first morning, she asked me what I wanted for breakfast, I asked for some bacon and eggs, and she got up to make it. It felt weird when she did. I was already uncomfortable with what I felt was the elitism and privilege of being at such an expensive place. Both in my personal life and in my career, I've never felt great about being waited on. Don't get me wrong, I'm super grateful that I've had people helping me take care of things in my life for many years, but they are nearly always on the payroll. I'm talking about the act and spirit of *service*. When someone *wants* to take care of you. That was far more foreign to me. And while this may have been Beth's job, she was doing it because she really wanted to. And though I've always felt that the reason I didn't like being served by others is because I always strive to stay real and grounded, that's only part of the truth. What's also true, I've come to learn, is that I wasn't comfortable with it because I didn't really know how to receive it well. I wasn't good at that. I didn't know how to be healthily mothered. I didn't have enough practice. Growing up, I never had real, consistent, healthy parenting. I'd had to learn to take care of myself, and it's taken me a long time to learn that it's okay to need some mothering. It's okay to need to be taken care of sometimes. Starting that morning, and over the course of the following weeks, I started to piece together why it was so important for this place to have all these services provided, because they were taking care of people like me who can barely get out of bed, who are barely able to take care of themselves. When I relaxed and allowed myself to receive it, it felt quite warm to have somebody doing the normal, everyday things that a mom would do.

Once Beth finished making breakfast, she brought it over and sat with me while I ate. We talked some more, and there was something about her, something about her presence, that made me feel okay to unburden myself a bit. She was graceful and calm and gentle, and I could tell she was full of the deepest empathy. I started unloading about why I was there and what I'd been going through and how I was feeling. Then I mentioned that I planned on going to church while I was there, that I had seen some options of different churches in the area, and I'd decided to visit The Vineyard. Her eyes lit up. "Oh, what a small world," she said. "That's my church! My husband's the pastor."

It was, in hindsight, a truly remarkable moment. I knew that I felt an immediate connection with her, but I didn't yet know what that connection would mean. What I didn't know was that this kind and gentle woman sitting across the breakfast table from me would be the one to bring me back from the abyss, that God would use her to help save my life—that she was, without question, an angel sent from heaven.

Ultimately, by the time I left Connecticut, I would truly want to live again, but for the moment I was still stuck in my head. I was still coming at everything from an intellectual standpoint. I'd come to this place in search of answers, solutions, a mental health to-do list with action items that I could check off. My engineer's mind wanted to know how things worked, what was broken, and how I could get under the hood and fix it.

One reason losing my faith in God had hit me so hard was that my whole life I've been adamant that there is, there *has to be*, some form of objective truth. Some objective truths are obvious, like gravity. Gravity doesn't need you to believe in it in order for it to work. It's gravity. It just works. But there are other truths, too, such as "It's better to be kind than not be kind." To me that's objective truth. It's a universal principle. The difference is you *do* have to believe that being kind is better than not being kind in order to see that it works. You have to manifest it in your actions. But people don't always treat those types of truths as universal. "Everything's relative," they say, and everything that cannot be scientifically proven or measured gets put into this category of "Well, that's your truth and this is my truth." Which has always driven me completely insane, because applying subjectivity erodes the objectivity of hard, constant, actual truth.

One of the issues I started to work out in Connecticut is where this rigidity of mine came from. I think in large part it has to do with my not being parented in a healthy or productive way. My mother in particular was so volatile, I was forever in a state of trying to figure out which side of her was going to be on display in any given moment and how I was supposed to relate to her. "There *has* to be an answer to this riddle," young Zac would tell himself, subconsciously. "There *has* to be a correct way to behave that solves this problem and keeps me away from the wrath and insanity of my mom." So I became obsessed with finding it.

Ultimately, in the absence of proper parenting, I found those rules and that truth in God, in the Bible. "This is the handbook," I was taught. "These are God's step-by-step instructions for living a good and worthy life." Amazing. Wonderful. I'll take that. And that sustained me for a long time. But now that my faith had crumbled, I was at a complete loss for how to orient myself in a world with no objective truth. Had I spent my whole life toeing the line of a Christianity that isn't even real? And if it isn't real, then what are the rules? What is the objective truth of how to live a good and worthy life? The thought of not knowing terrified me.

Having lost my faith, I was flying without a compass. I had lost my true north. Because of that, I was frantically looking for a new set of step-by-step instructions from medical science itself. I arrived in Connecticut with unrealistic expectations of what they could do for me. I was incredibly eager to sit down with the psychiatrist, because the job of a psychiatrist is to assess your mental health from a medical point of view. To me, he was the guy who could give me the capital-D diagnosis that nobody else had been able to provide. I was hungry for those answers. I was desperate for them.

> Finding the right therapist is crucial. I would add that sometimes, *sometimes*, we don't feel like a therapist is the right fit merely because they might actually be *great* at their job, and we don't like how closely they might be hitting on the truth.

For that same reason, I was frustrated in my sessions with the psychotherapist. Psychotherapy is all that emotional, Kleenexy, "Tell me about your childhood" kind of stuff. Psychotherapy is where you vent. You're dredging up all the trauma and pain and regurgitating it, puking it up, getting it all out. Hopefully, you're having breakthroughs while you're getting it all out. But by and large you sit there and the doctor keeps saying, "Soooo, tell me about your father . . ." and "Soooo, how did that make you *feel* . . . ?" Meanwhile, you're sitting there, like, *What's the* fucking point *of this? When are you going to tell me what's* wrong *with me?*

That was my attitude, 100 percent, and from the jump, there were really only two questions I wanted answers to. The first was "How did I end up here?" and the second was "How do I never end up here again?" Specifically, I wanted to know if I had a condition. Was I just a broken, traumatized person struggling with the same shit that every broken, traumatized person goes through, or did I have an actual, diagnosable physiological condition that was ruining my life that I needed to know about?

My sisters and I had always suspected my mom might have been bipolar. Possibly our grandfather too. We were also keenly aware of the possibility that the condition could be hereditary. For a while, Shekinah had been 100 percent convinced that I was bipolar too. She's seen a lot of my ups and downs, and she cares about me and is a bit of a worrier. When she was booking me into Connecticut and doing all the intake processing, she straight-up told them: "I think Zac may be bipolar."

And look, I had no idea if I was bipolar or not. I knew that I had my ups and downs, and I knew that my highs could get pretty high and my lows could get *really* low, but I had also started reading and researching everything about mental health I could put my hands on, and by that point I'd read enough to know that my symptoms didn't necessarily correlate with bipolarity. My ups and downs seemed to be precipitated by events, rather than randomly shifting chemicals in my brain. And the typical up-down cycle of someone who's bipolar tends to run in relatively short spurts, super high for three weeks, then plummeting down down down for a week, and then back up again for another few weeks, and so on and so forth. My highs could last for months, and they always correlated to my feeling that other people valued me, whether it was a new girlfriend or a new job. My lows could also last for months and months, and they always correlated with not working or breaking up or an overall lack of self-confidence.

Still, there was evidence pointing the other way as well. The psychiatrist I saw briefly in Austin told me that in certain instances of bipolarity, you see the world in a different way because at times 25 percent of your brain is firing, as opposed to the 5 percent in "normal" brain activity. This seemed familiar to how I felt a lot of the time because of the way I've struggled with my mind feeling like it's in hyperactive overdrive much of the time. I told myself,

*Hey, if you're going to have a debilitating mental illness, at least it's cool to be some kind of mad genius because your brain is working too well.* So I was doing my best to make peace with the idea of being bipolar, if in fact that was my reality. Mostly, I just wanted to know what the fuck my reality was.

As far as ensuring that I never ended up back in this place again, I also wanted answers about medication—even though I already knew the answer I wanted to hear. I wanted them to tell me, "You don't need it." Because I didn't want it. One of the few positives of my mother's parenting was her insistence on organic foods and holistic health. Back in the eighties, there were administrators at my school who suggested that I be put on Ritalin because I was super hyperactive, bouncing off the walls and kooky all the time. My mom, to

> Dig in and surround yourself with people who want to dig in with you and force you to be better.

her credit, said no. I was grateful for that, and as an adult I've continued to be the same way. I never wanted to admit that I needed a pill to get my mind right. But then I kept running into these issues that I was having, and I'd started to face the reality that maybe I wouldn't have a choice.

Six months before, while I was still living in LA, I had a friend with an Adderall prescription. It helped them a lot when it came to managing their life and remembering details and whatnot. I'd used it recreationally when going to parties here and there, as some people do, but never consistently for its intended purpose. So I finally decided to try it. The truth is it was one of the most fascinating things that has ever happened to me. One of my biggest problems has always been that I don't feel capable of tackling the chaos in my life. There were too many unresolved issues floating around, too much to do, and I would always find myself paralyzed by them. But with Adderall, I found myself waking up in the morning and instead of being sluggish and overwhelmed and defeated and despondent, I felt capable and confident and optimistic about my day. It was like somebody had flipped a switch.

Which should come as no surprise, as Adderall is an amphetamine, and like all amphetamines what it does is supercharge the activity of dopamine in our system. Dopamine is our reward and encouragement hormone. Dopamine makes us feel like we can take on the next challenge, and the next, and the next, and the next. It helps us feel capable of tackling and accomplishing the little, medium, and big tasks that are in our every day. So did Adderall actually make me a better, more productive person? Was it a magic pill that made everything better? No. But it definitely helped the reward system in my body work competently enough to get me out of a rut and moving forward.

My intention was never to stay on it forever, just to see if it would help me out. I was still very much against medication as any kind of permanent crutch, and I stopped taking it before I moved to Texas. Then, after the Chi'Lantro incident, I was at my wit's end from trying to figure out a way to not feel so sad and crazy all the time, and I finally broke down and agreed to let my local Austin psychiatrist prescribe me Lexapro, an antidepressant, and carbamazepine, which is typically used as an anti-seizure medication. Because if I were bipolar and prone to having an overactive brain, the medication would help to quell the frantic firing of my synapses.

It takes about a month for any of those drugs to start having an effect. By the time I got to Connecticut, I'd been on them a few weeks and I wasn't sure they were even doing anything.

I didn't want to be putting them in my body any longer than I had to, and the first thing I asked the psychiatrist when I got to Connecticut was, "Do I keep taking these drugs or not? Is this the wrong thing to be taking? Is there something else I should be taking?"

To which he replied, "We don't know what you should be taking yet, so just keep taking it."

Which drove me nuts, to be honest, because (a) it was not an actual answer, (b) he was the guy I was expecting to give me an actual answer, and (c) taking drugs not even knowing what kind of effect they'll have seems . . . kind of crazy!

Because of my own fears and rigidity, I struggled in a lot of my early sessions, especially the ones like art therapy. I would get frustrated because I suck at drawing, and really, what was the point of it? What was I doing? How was this getting me any closer to the answers I was seeking? I didn't need to be scribbling on construction paper with crayons like I was in elementary school.

In other words, I was doing it wrong. I was so fixated on what I wanted that I wasn't being open to what I needed. Because of that my first week was incredibly difficult. Practically every session felt like a psychotherapy session, which was the opposite of what I'd had in mind. Every session was me introducing myself to this yet-again new person and having to tell them my whole life story, all the way from Grandma Pat and her butcher knife up through bawling my eyes out in the Chi'Lantro parking lot. I had to go through my crazy tale of woe with every single one of the specialists and pretty soon I felt like I had talked myself to death. It was beyond frustrating. I don't know why there couldn't have been one big group session where I gave everyone the same spiel at the same time, and then they could divvy it up from there. But that wasn't how they did it. They wanted me to go from session to session and vomit up the same story over and over again.

So that's what I did.

# FOUR

# Look Behind You

Emotional trauma can be generational, passed down from parent to child like a family heirloom. You carry it with you and it's not even yours.

. . .

To understand the root of all my struggles with mental health, picture a glass of water. It's sitting on the kitchen counter, glistening with condensation as the ice inside it crackles and melts on a hot summer day. Six years old and all rambunctious and sweaty from running around in the yard, I run into the house to get a drink and, being a hyper kid and bit of a spaz, I knock the glass over and it shatters across the kitchen floor.

Now, if I knock that glass over and my mom is in a good mood, she'll turn from whatever she's doing and say, sweet as can be, "Oh honey, it's okay. Don't worry about it. We can get another glass." But if I knock that glass over and she's in a bad mood, she'll turn on me and scream, "*Look what you did, you little shit! What the fuck is wrong with you?! You fucking idiot!*"

That was my mother: rational, kind, and loving—or irrational, volatile, and lashing out in anger at the slightest provocation. Living with her was like living with Jekyll and Hyde, and on any given day, my sisters and I had no idea which way she was going to go, what would set her off, or how far it would escalate. The glass of water could be anything: a fight with my sisters, a bad grade on a test, playing the radio too loud. It could be something supremely important, or something completely trivial; it didn't matter. We were forever walking on eggshells and dodging trip mines. Throw in her ever-increasing alcohol dependency and the slowly deteriorating codependent relationship with my equally broken and abusive stepdad, and the rest of the script writes itself. It wasn't unusual to come home to find all of my stepdad's shit on the front lawn because my mom had decided to throw it out there. It was just as typical to come home and find all my mom's shit out on the lawn because my stepdad had decided it was his turn to do the same. There was nothing remarkable or special about any of it. Coming home to some kind of emotional Armageddon was like, "Oh, it's Tuesday."

My sisters and I were being traumatized, plain and simple. It wasn't blunt-force physical trauma; we weren't getting beaten by our parents, thank God, but we were getting psychologically KO'd on a daily basis. For the longest time, I didn't know that it was abnormal. I assumed that this was how everybody's parents were, that this was how human beings operated. And because I thought it was normal, I couldn't see the negative effects it was having, or how those negative effects were accumulating and compounding in my head, year after year after year. Once I became an adult, I couldn't see the ways in which I still approached every aspect of my life the way I did that glass of water: terrified that anything other than perfection would trigger an onslaught of pain and abuse and rejection.

Still, my mother was not a bad, or evil, person. In fact, she naturally had deep empathy and love for people, and a desire to do good things in the world. But her natural inclinations wound up being overridden all too often because she was a damaged person and, ultimately, a broken person, and when I set out to learn why, to answer the question behind the glass of water, I didn't have to look too hard to find the culprit; it's right there in the family tree, in the long history of unwellness that goes back not just to my mom but far into my extended family as well.

If you found yourself suffering from a debilitating condition, like heart disease or breast cancer, what's one of the first things you would you do? You'd go to your family tree. You'd look back to see where it mostly likely came from in order to narrow down the root causes and the best course of treatment. With the advances in DNA analysis we have now, it's amazing what science can do. Mental health is no different. The root causes are all there. You just have to go looking for them. Needless to say, not every trauma or condition is linked to family. You may suffer from trauma at work or be in an abusive relationship, but if your story is anything like mine, a lot of your answers are tucked away with the skeletons in the family closet.

Trying to figure out your family history is a journey, and a tough one at that. Getting people to open up about the trauma they've endured is not an easy thing to do. People are often unwilling to talk. Or, if they do talk, they're unwilling to be honest. Everyone is doing their best to frame the past the way they want to see it, which is not necessarily the way that it actually was. Still, you do the best you can. You become a bit of an archaeologist. You search and you dig, and ultimately you piece together facts and form conclusions from the best evidence you can gather. Which is why you start by telling your own story. You regurgitate all the unhealthy patterns and behaviors you witnessed and endured over the years, and that at least gives you a place to start. But the cool thing is that by understanding psychology more, by going to therapy more, by learning about yourself more, you in turn learn so much about your parents and your family—and the world, for that matter.

I wish more than anything that I'd had someone in my life when I was younger to help guide me and heal myself. Nearly all of our collective woes on earth can be traced back to the broken hearts and minds of people.

With my mother's story, the evidence I have to go on is largely anecdotal. She didn't leave a paper trail. She never once went to a therapist, never once sought any kind of help or treatment for her problems, except when she was ordered to by the court to avoid jail time. So there's no formal diagnosis, no medical file full of patient notes and assessments. But after talking to multiple therapists now about my own issues, telling them the basic scenarios about what my mom was like, the near-unanimous conclusion is that my mom was a classic borderline personality with narcissistic tendencies, meaning her personality and demeanor could change on a dime and she had to be right all the time. There's some conjecture that she was bipolar as well, but there's no way of knowing that for sure without a proper diagnosis.

Of course, any attempt to map out the trauma in your family tree will bring you quickly to the question of nature versus nurture. Were we born this way, or was something done to us? My understanding is that the mood swings that come with being bipolar are rooted in biology, in hormones and genetics. Being a borderline personality, on the other hand, is a condition spawned by trauma and abuse. Trying to tease out the difference between the two can be difficult. How much of this generational relay race is genetic, and how much of it is learned behavior that we take on by growing up in proximity to unhealthy people?

> I personally believe that trauma from our nurture quite literally reprograms our nature, even chromosomally.

Scientifically, we know that at least some of it is nature. We know that there are certain chromosomes and the way they line up and how they switch on and off can affect your body and your emotions in all number of ways. We also know that your environment, and a traumatic environment in particular, can have a profound effect on the physical development of the brain, activating different genes and shaping different neural pathways, exacerbating preexisting genetic issues, and ingraining unhealthy behaviors that can take a lifetime to correct.

And I will say, after all the learning I've done, the answer lies somewhere in the middle. It is both nature and nurture. That said, my personal feelings about what caused my mother's problems— as well as my problems and the problems of the vast majority of people on earth—lean toward nurture. Perhaps I'm biased that way because of what I've been through. Perhaps I'm biased that way because I'm a person who wants to believe in solutions, and if the problem is how we nurture each other, then that means we have the power to do better. And if we have the power to help each other, to love each other, to help heal each other, then we can do it right now. And maybe I want to believe that if someone had been able to do those things for my mother, if someone had been able to halt the cycle of generational abuse before it inflicted so much damage on her, then maybe, just maybe, she wouldn't have died alone on her bathroom floor, never knowing how much her friends and family truly loved her.

My mother was born Susan Marie Hoctor in 1950 in St. Louis, Missouri. She was the oldest of five, with two sisters, Sally and Sandy, and two brothers, Tim and Mike—five children born in seven years to one of those big Catholic families that used to pop them out like that back then. My maternal grandfather, Grandpa Ed, was a psychiatrist, ironically, and when my mom was young, he moved the family to Ventura, California, so he could take a job at Camarillo State Hospital, which had one of the preeminent psych wards on the West Coast. Grandpa Ed was super smart, well educated, and successful.

Then there was Grandma Pat.

The Grandma Pat stories are legendary. I mean, she was a tyrant, a ballbuster extraordinaire, strictly and oppressively Catholic but also extremely volatile, always yelling and screaming and abusing in one form or another. One story that my mom and her siblings used to tell all the time was about when my mom was twelve and the family was driving across the country. My mom was being more mouthy than Grandma Pat felt was proper, so as they passed by some truck stop in the middle of nowhere, Grandma Pat kicked her out of the car and left her there, for a half an hour, a twelve-year-old girl at a truck stop, by herself, surrounded by strangers, just to teach her a lesson.

All of Grandma Pat's kids are around the same age, share the same DNA, grew up in the same insanely disruptive home, and struggle with the consequences. To this day I'm not sure any of them have fully reckoned with it. Nobody's sure why Grandma Pat was such a tyrant, because supposedly her mom and dad were quite kind, but part of it might have had something to do with the fact that Grandpa Ed was gay. He lived his whole life in the closet, hiding it from his family, because of how difficult it was for a gay man to live openly in those times. He and Grandma Pat had five kids, and they slept together probably five times. Grandma Pat used to come home and find him socializing late into the night with other men, having drinks. Ignorance is bliss and she didn't want to believe it, so for a while Grandpa Ed was just considered eccentric and cosmopolitan. But eventually she caught him red-handed and the façade of the marriage crumbled around them. Grandma Pat was stuck raising the kids by herself for eight years until she remarried, but I think the whole experience unhinged her a bit, as I imagine it would with anyone.

I didn't know my Grandpa Ed at all. He moved up to Santa Maria after that. The only time I can remember visiting him was when he was living with his "roommate" Buzz. Not his boyfriend, his *roommate*—a very Bert-and-Ernie type of situation. Then, when I was around seven or so, I came home one day and there was a box with all this random stuff in it, board games and VHS tapes and this cool robot that had a controller with a walkie-talkie so you could move it around and talk out of its speaker. It was like Christmas morning!

"What's all this?!" I asked.

"Your grandfather died," my mom said, "and he gave you all that."

"Great!"

I wasn't even fazed. It's sad, but I genuinely didn't know the man, and I had no comprehension of what had happened. I only learned the details much later, that after years of struggling with his own mental health issues, he drank NyQuil for three weeks straight until it killed him.

If there's one thing that everyone in our family agrees on, it's that my mom was the smartest, prettiest, and most charismatic of the bunch. She graduated from high school in 1968, and she could have done anything she wanted. She could have had a successful business or run for governor. She had that power in her; that much was undeniable. But being an eighteen-year-old girl fleeing an abusive home in Southern California in the late sixties, it was practically preordained that she become a hippie. So that's what she did. She left Ventura for a quick stint at a Santa Barbara City College, then dropped out, moved to Los Angeles, and never went back to finish.

> Trauma may be generational, but so is enlightenment. We have such an amazing opportunity to break down the chains of abuse, the chains of trauma, the chains of shame and fear and insecurity and ignorance and lack of understanding and all of it.

At the time, the whole hippie-Jesus movement was taking off, so my mom started gravitating toward that, rejecting the dogma and stigma of the Catholicism she'd grown up with her whole life. After a few years of bouncing around Southern California embracing her hippie-Jesus self, my mom started going to a church out in the San Fernando Valley called Church of the Living Word. It was there in 1976 that she met my dad, the new lead singer in the worship band, who'd recently moved to LA after eight years in the Air Force. My dad was this hunky, six-foot-three seventies dude with long hair and a big Grizzly Adams beard. But while my dad had the outward appearance of this burly, bearded man's man, inside he was mostly a nerdy, insecure kid dealing with generational trauma of his own (which we'll get to later on).

Ultimately, my parents were two broken people who grabbed onto each other to feel less broken, with predictable results. "I was just a simple Indiana boy who got caught up in the California cyclone who was your mother," my dad always says, and boy he ain't lying.

The tragic irony is that my mother became this free-spirited hippie because she wanted to rebel against the life she'd grown up with. She wanted to do better and be better than Grandma Pat. But trauma, if unacknowledged and untreated, will always get passed on. And because my mother had never done the work to understand and heal the abuse she'd grown up with, she fell right back into acting out the script she knew. She rejected a home with a domineering, abusive mother and a passive, emotionally cloistered father, only to run away and re-create that exact scenario for herself and her children.

Second verse, same as the first.

# FIVE

# Tell Your Story

*You are not yourself. You are the story you tell yourself about yourself.
And as the author of that story, you have the power to rewrite the ending.*

. . .

Human beings love stories. Books, podcasts, television shows, movies—we devour them. It's something that's universal across cultures. It's been a constant from the days of tribal peoples recounting their greatest adventures on cave walls up to the latest streaming series you're watching on your phone. It's the reason why Hollywood is the global behemoth it is. It's the reason why actors like me have the job that we do. We exist to tell stories.

If you've never stopped to ask yourself why, the answer is because the human brain is wired for it. We are storytelling animals because stories are the mechanism through which we store and process information. Think about what happens when someone asks you where you were born. You might give them a one-word answer, but more than likely you're going to tell them your origin story: the town where you were born, why your parents lived there at the time, what your parents did, how long you lived there before you moved away, why you moved away, and so on. Because all those facts are stored in a narrative sequence, and it is the narrative sequence that gives the facts meaning. A good story takes a fact and gives it direction and momentum—a trajectory. The stories we tell ourselves in common, the myths and legends spun by political leaders and others, become the organizing forces of the culture that shapes us as a society, for good and for ill. Meanwhile, the personal stories we tell ourselves about ourselves become the dominant forces that shape how we perceive our own lives, also for good and for ill.

As much as I didn't love the weepy, navel-gazing regurgitation of psychotherapy, I have to acknowledge that it served its purpose during my time in Connecticut. Telling your story in the presence of a therapist—or, for that matter, a good book editor—is a cathartic process. Because you don't simply tell your story. You interrogate it. You challenge it. You put the facts down in cold black and white and you go back over them again and again, forcing yourself to see the ways in which you've been mischaracterizing and even lying to yourself about major events of your life. You recast those events in a different light based on your new understanding of yourself, and, almost magically, the story of a hopeless young romantic who couldn't get his shit together becomes the story of a man approaching middle age, humbled by his own failures and moving forward with self-love and self-acceptance. You rewrite your own story as it's happening, and the tragic ending that seemed so inevitable can change into something completely amazing and new.

I was born on September 29, 1980, in Lake Charles, Louisiana. That fact alone tells you nothing. But the story behind it tells you everything, and the story is that my parents had gotten married and had my older sister, Sarah, a few years before. At the time, my dad worked for an industrial robotic welding equipment manufacturer, the same company he would work for his entire life. He was one of their technicians, and part of his job was to go on location at the factories and power plants that used this welding equipment, to instruct their workers on how to operate these complicated machines. Sometimes he'd stay for months to make sure everything was working correctly. Since he got paid better for those location jobs, and because my mom liked to travel, they were nomads for a while, living in different cities all over the country. Which is how I came to be born in a small town in Southern Louisiana. It was a fluke. I have no connection to the place; it's just where my parents happened to be when I popped out.

Most of my earliest memories start in Nebraska, another random place we lived when I was three. I remember getting a *Star Wars* blaster gun and a He-Man bicycle for Christmas and being stoked, but I think the main reason Nebraska sticks out in my memory is because, for my parents, Nebraska was essentially the beginning of the end: more screaming, more fighting, more walking out and not being home for bedtime.

My real home was always back in Ventura, California, where my mom's family was from and where my little sister, Shekinah, was born three years later. By the time we landed back in Ventura full-time, my parent's marriage was completely on the rocks. They were fighting like cats and dogs, to the point where it was frightening to me. I remember, vividly, being four or five years old and throwing myself into the middle of a heated exchange. They were right up in each other's faces, and I ran, pushed myself in between them, tears in my eyes, grabbing onto their legs and begging, "Please don't fight. Please don't yell at each other." That time it actually worked. They both looked down at me, and they stopped, as if they realized for the first time that all of this insanity was affecting their children. But then the next time I did it, they kept on yelling. The trick didn't work anymore. Their disdain for one another and their unhappiness had so consumed them that they were completely desensitized to the pain they were inflicting on my sisters and me.

The only relief from the fighting came when my dad would leave to go back on the road for work again, which he had to do to keep up with the massive credit card bills my mom was racking up. In truth, I think part of the reason we settled down in one place was because my mother no longer wanted to travel with my dad, and my dad was happy to have work as his excuse to be gone. There were at least a couple of years when they were still married but he always had one foot out the door on his way to someplace else. My mom would scream at him, accusing him of running away and not dealing with their marriage, at which point he would, essentially, slip away as fast as he could in order to not deal with their marriage.

I honestly can't even tell you when my dad "left" because it was such a slow fade. He was gone on this trip and that trip, and then he took one trip and didn't come back. They filed for divorce, and my dad moved up to Placerville, California, near Lake Tahoe, where his job had relocated. We stayed behind in Ventura with our mom. We'd see him on weekends here and there, and for a few weeks in the summer, but otherwise we were three small kids being raised by a marginally employed, emotionally volatile single mother.

And you know what? Those were the salad days. I'm not kidding. They actually were. It may not sound great, being strung between a mentally ill mother and a perpetually absent father. But compared to what came after, those elementary school years were the happiest of my childhood. That was in part, I think, because those were the years when my mother was happiest. Every time she was pregnant, she was happy. Every time she had a baby, she was happy, at least for a while. She had these little creatures to snuggle and hold and take care of. And she did, in her own way, do her best to raise us well. Her demons and darkness hadn't evolved into their full form yet; that would come with time. Moreover, she really did care about our well-being. She was way ahead of the curve when it came to nutrition and eating organic fruits and vegetables and whole-grain barley and wheatgrass and all that stuff that's trendy nowadays. We were raised taking vitamins and supplements and never had sugared cereal or sugared soda. She instilled good habits in us that I carry to this day.

My mom also ran with a fun crowd. Her hippie days were behind her by that point, and she had entered what you might call her 1980s hair-band era. She knew a lot of free spirits in the music scene down in LA. She'd leave us with a sitter and go down to see shows at all the spots on the Sunset Strip. In fact, for a while she even worked as the assistant to ZZ Top's road manager. She was always showing up with random people: roadies, groupies, drummers, local Ventura rock guys, and they'd hang out at the house. They were our buddies. For a kid, that was pretty fucking cool.

My mom also instilled in us a genuine drive to be good people, to be spiritual, to reach out to others and help them. For someone who could be unbelievably cruel to the people around her, my mom had an amazing ability to empathize with the less fortunate. I think that's something you see a lot of the time: broken people reaching out to people who are more broken than they are as a way to make themselves feel less broken. My mom was forever helping people who were lost, whether it was a friend from some rock band who needed a place to crash or a homeless person she'd met downtown that needed some help.

All in all, life was okay. My stepdad hadn't entered the picture, so that whole codependent death spiral had yet to begin. I missed my dad, but I was used to missing my dad, so it didn't seem that big of a deal. I just assumed we were normal. Even when I started going to other kids' houses and could see their moms doing "totally normal" mom things and not screaming and losing their shit all the time, I still thought we were like them, because when friends came over to my house, at least early on, my mom would be on far better behavior; she didn't like other people seeing her dirty laundry. I knew my mom would put on a face and do the mom thing whenever witnesses were around, so when I went over to friends' houses, I assumed their moms were doing the same thing. I assumed that all other families were lying and pretending too.

Which, let's be honest, a lot of families are.

So I was happy, as far as I knew. We lived in this cozy two-bedroom house. My mom had one bedroom, my sisters shared the other bedroom, and my room was the laundry room, which was great because I could fall asleep to the sound of the washer and dryer every night. I had lots of friends, too, from elementary school. One of our favorite things was finding half-built houses that were still under construction. We'd run around in the trenches that had been dug for the utility lines, grabbing dirt clods and chucking them at each other's faces. The worst thing that could have happened to us was that maybe some kid lost an eye, but nobody ever did. So we were always out of the house in the beautiful, warm Southern California weather, having a blast, running around the neighborhood barefoot at dusk, the pavement still warm under our feet. It was lovely. It was idyllic. And it would never be that way again.

I was nine years old when my stepdad, Gary, entered the picture. Gary was an architect and a musician. The story we were always told growing up was that he'd been a musical prodigy, playing the violin with the San Diego Symphony at the age of five, or something like that. Around the time he moved in with my mom, he was getting into digital audio production, dabbling in MIDI and Pro Audio; he knew everything there was to know at the time about music and computers. He was kind of a nerdy guy, tall and thin and pale with reddish-brown hair that he wore in kind of a mullet in the back, and sometimes a goatee in the front. Gary carried himself like a bit of a snooty intellectual a lot of the time, which didn't do him any favors. In fairness, he was a highly intelligent person in a lot of ways, but as with a lot of smart people, his brilliance often blinded him from seeing how awkward and unkind he really was a lot of the time. Unsurprisingly, Gary also had a generational trauma story of his own, having been raised by an abusive father himself.

I don't recall where or how he and my mom met; I just remember him sort of showing up and moving in after leaving his first wife and two kids to be with us. As far as I know, he and my mom were never technically, legally married; they were very much about keeping the government out of their personal lives and business. But they did have a whole spiritual ceremony with friends, and from that point on they lived together as husband and wife in the common-law sense. Gary moved in with us in Ventura, then soon after that he got a job offer in the Northwest and we relocated to Olympia, Washington, for a year before finally settling outside Seattle, where we lived in an apartment across the street from a little upstart tech company called Microsoft.

Moving to Seattle was the beginning of a dark, difficult period for me. It was the first time I went through what I can now recognize as clinical depression. I was this kid from sunny, beautiful Southern California, and all of a sudden I was transplanted up to this lonely place that was gray and overcast and rainy and wet ten months out of the year. In Ventura, I'd had the same crew of friends all through elementary school. Now I was a new kid, with no friends at all, and I was starting sixth grade. Sixth grade is the beginning of middle school—and middle school, holy fuck. In elementary school, kids are still kids, you know? It's not that hard to get along. Everyone has the same interests, which are snacks and recess. But middle school is when kids turn into real

> Our parents or family or friends or society may well begin the cycle of judgment in our lives, but we are the only ones responsible for or capable of fixing it deep within ourselves.

assholes. Because middle schoolers all want to be high schoolers, and high schoolers all want to be adults. All of a sudden, life turns into cliques and groups. It's all about having status, wearing the right kind of clothes, and having the right kind of gear. It's all about what's cool and what's not cool and who's cool and who's not cool. It's so weird and subjective, and it's all informed by what your older siblings think is cool, what the TV is saying is cool, and what your particular community and society at large are dictating is cool. Then you grow up and you realize that everything you thought was cool is not cool, or healthy in any way, shape, or form.

I was not cool. I was the spazzy, dorky theater kid on rollerblades—and that was not a good look. I was teased incessantly, mocked and made fun of and bullied on a daily basis by at least one if not multiple people. Let's start with the fact that my last name was Pugh, okay? Everybody made fun of that. They would make up rhymes about me: "Zachary daiquiri dock / ran up a grandfather clock. / The clock struck two and down he flew into a big bowl of poo." I mean, A for effort and all, but it sure wasn't fun for little Zac. And being the people pleaser I was, I was constantly trying to be friends with everybody and not be bullied. For a while I tried to lean into it. At one point in seventh grade, I gave myself the nickname "Stinky," hoping that if I joked about it first then the other kids wouldn't be so harsh. So dumb. Didn't work.

There was this thing that kids did then called "backjazzing," which was where they would make a fist with a knuckle sticking out, come up behind you, and then punch you as hard as they could in the middle of your spine. This one kid, Tom, who made up the "fun" rhymes, used to do that to me all the time. He and his friends would all get off on it and laugh about it, endlessly.

One time, when the bell rang at the end of my second-period class, I got up, put on my backpack, and walked through the halls to my third-period class. When I got there, I took my backpack off, set it on my desk, and there, planted on the outside pocket, was a massive fresh loogie that somebody had hocked on my back as I was walking through the hallways, the snot and spit still gooey and gelatinous.

Shit like that happened *daily*, and because my parents had no idea how to handle situations like these without somehow making them worse, I was covering it all up, maintaining this happy, funny-guy façade, pretending everything was fine even as the storm clouds in my brain started to grow dark and ominous. All of a sudden, I felt alone. I didn't have a safe place to go. I was very much by myself. I had a few friends, but none of them were capable of being my confidants. I had my sisters, but I wouldn't say the three of us were close. Today we are; we're in the best shape we've ever been as far as our family dynamic is concerned. We've all watched our family deteriorate; they've seen me go through my mental health challenges, and I think that's opened their eyes to their own mental health needs. We've all started to work on ourselves and we've grown enough to finally come together. But that wasn't the case back then. Back then Sarah wanted to hang out with her older, cooler high school friends, not her goofy brother who was the last person you would ever bring around people you were trying to impress. Shekinah and I were closer. With her I could be cool just by being older, and we could hang out and watch cartoons and play video games. But collectively, the three of us weren't able to articulate what we were going through, so we couldn't talk to each other and protect each other. In some families, abuse can bring siblings closer together, but in our family, for a long time, it served to isolate us and push us apart. None of us was trying to hurt each other, but I think we all wanted to get out of the house and away from the family to grab onto some kind of life preserver to keep us afloat in the storm. It was survival, plain and simple.

We didn't have other adults around to help or protect us either. Moving to the Northwest had sealed the deal on my ever having any kind of relationship with my father. Around the time my mom and Gary decided to move, my dad's job was relocating to Charlotte, North Carolina, and my dad reasoned, "Well, if she's taking them to Seattle, I won't be able to see them but once a year anyway, so I'm going to go ahead and follow this job across the country." From then on we only saw him once a year. For a couple of weeks every summer he'd come up to Washington and, weirdly, stay with us in our home with our mom and our stepdad, which was *sooooooo* fucking strange.

Anyone with divorced parents can attest to the bizarreness of having them under the same roof at holidays and other occasions. For us, it was made infinitely stranger by the way our mother was always attempting to program our young minds about who our dad was or was not. Even years after the divorce, he was still one of her most used scapegoats. She used to rail on him all year long. I don't think she ever went more than a few weeks without talking about (a) what a bastard he was, (b) how he didn't love us, (c) how he'd deserted us, and (d) how he was "such a fucking pussy." Though not always in that order. Then my dad would show up to live with us for two weeks and everyone would pretend that all the shit-talking from the other fifty weeks of the year had never happened. Inevitably, some massive fight would break out and she'd start yelling all that shit directly to his face right in front of us. This would be followed by an hour of more insanity and vitriol, after which my dad would disappear and curl up in bed on my bottom bunk. It was weird, and not a good weird. It wasn't "odd." It was profoundly unhealthy.

Other than those visits, my dad and I mostly talked every Sunday on the phone for five minutes or so, doing what he called "swappin' howdies."

"Hey, Dad."

"Hey, son. Just swappin' howdies. How you doin'?"

"Good. How you doin', Dad?"

"Oh, y'know, better than I deserve. God is good."

"Okay, cool."

We might as well have been talking about the weather.

My stepdad wasn't someone I could turn to either. Now, I had some respect for Gary as someone who'd stepped in to be the breadwinner for three kids who weren't his, and I always tried to give him a bit of the benefit of the doubt because of that. But there was no warmth to the guy. Moreover, where my mom's love and approval were difficult to attain due to her constantly shifting emotional target, Gary's love and approval sat at the top of an unscalable summit of perfectionism. Perfectionism that wreaked havoc on me and my sisters, and still has lingering effects to this day. In fact, they might even tell you that Gary's actions caused them more damage than my mom's. Each of us went through the same fire but have different scars to show for it.

My sisters and I were taught no discipline either. My mom was all over the place when it came to our behavior. Discipline to her was screaming and flying off the handle and making you feel horrible by calling you a stupid little shit. She'd say all the right stuff, like "I'll ground you for a month" or "No more TV!" But we learned quickly that all you had to do was play the game, crawl back to her, and give her a quick "I'm sorry, Mommy. I love you, Mommy," and lo and behold, she'd forget about whatever it was. There were never any real consequences beyond how horrible she'd make you feel in the beginning. We never actually got grounded, the TV never actually got taken away, so we never learned anything.

Sometimes Gary would come in and try to drop the hammer and we'd give him an earful of "You're not my dad! You can't tell me what to do!" When that happened, our mom would take our side against Gary. So we didn't listen to him at all. Other than paying the bills, Gary was quickly a parent in name only. He was neither an authority figure you obeyed nor a mentor you'd go to for advice or emotional support. The only bit of warmth I had in our childhood was when my mom was in a good mood, and as time went on the good moods became increasingly hard to come by.

My mom did to my sisters and me exactly what Grandma Pat had done to her. My mom also grew up in a home with a glass of water perched precariously on the edge of the counter. If she did anything wrong, the immediate reaction from her mother was, "You *idiot*! You *dummy*!" Which meant my mother could never be wrong if she wanted to please Grandma Pat. In order to be loved, my mom had to be right. That was the fire in which my mother was forged. That was the programming that allowed her to survive a tyrant like Grandma Pat.

Out in the world, however, that programming didn't serve her well. You can't always be right and still have healthy relationships that are built on communication and sharing and compromise and vulnerability. So as my mom got older, never understanding how and why her neural pathways had been so damaged by trauma, she could never admit that she was wrong about anything; deep down she believed that being wrong meant not being worthy of being loved. But where my dad was meek and mostly rolled over and ran away from my mom, Gary could be as stubborn as she was. I think it had something to do with him being a musical prodigy as a kid; you don't become a prodigy violinist without some task-master standing over you, cracking the whip to make you think you have to be flawless and perfect all the time. So together, Gary and my mom were unbelievably unhealthy and codependent. They used to have these long knockdown, drag-out fights. Gary punched copious holes in several walls. Big shocker: they both drank a lot.

Their fights all started like most married-people fights do, with one person communicating poorly and the other person respond-ing poorly to that poor communication. What started as a snipe or quip about nothing would build and build and build, escalating to the point where they would say or do anything to dehumanize and degrade each other. It was always, "You're a worthless bastard!" and every other insult in the book. At some point, they'd usually throw us kids under the bus. "Your kids *hate* you. You think your kids *like* you? They fucking *hate* you." Then it would invariably end in a hailstorm of threats, like "I'll leave you right now, mother-fucker!" and "I'll report you to the fucking government!" They would do this at restaurants, too, with one of them eventually storming out, taking the car, and leaving the other to figure out how to get home. I can't even tell you how many times I cried my-self to sleep, terrified, not knowing how bad things might get.

The same dynamic even extended to my mom and her siblings. Holidays were a fucking trip. Thanksgivings and Christmases were often at Grandma Pat's back in Ventura—my mom and her sib-lings, who'd all been abused, coming back together in the home of the abuser. Which they all still felt compelled to do, because when you've been abused by someone, unless you go do the deep therapy to either sever or fix that relationship, you'll keep going back to them, because that's the only programming you know. Tale as old as time.

For my mom, the holidays were an opportunity to play all sides. For weeks leading up to Christmas, she'd be at home talking to my stepdad about how abusive her family had been. Then she'd be on the phone with her family, telling all of them about what a dick Gary was. Then we'd all show up to celebrate the birth of Christ, and my mom would get to watch everyone go at each other, and feel everyone defending her against something somebody else had supposedly done to her. It always ended with everybody drinking too much and yelling and screaming about some shit from the past and somebody storming out. I was a kid watching all this hap-pen, but even then, I could see what my mom was doing. I was like, "This is *insane.*"

What I see now is that my mom needed those fights, because when she was being fought over, she was at least being recognized. I think one of the hardest things for my mom was that she felt like her pain wasn't acknowledged, which to a large degree was a legiti-mate gripe. To the bitter end, my Grandma Pat never apologized for, never even admitted, that any abuse had taken place in her home, and to the extent that she acknowledged any difficulty at all, it was always, "Well, I was totally justified in what I was doing, so I'm not going to apologize."

My sisters and I never acknowledged our mother's pain either. By the time we came of age, Grandma Pat had been through treatment for breast cancer; she'd had a mastectomy and chemo and radiation, which mellowed her out a bit. So, as horrible as she'd been to her own kids, she wasn't all that bad to us. My mom *hated* Grandma Pat. She was forever telling us how atrocious she had been. But, as kids, we didn't really understand that. We never witnessed the abuse inflicted on our mom, only the abuse that our mom inflicted on us. So we'd sit there and listen to our mom go off about her mother, and in our minds we were always like, *Yeah, okay. Sure. But at least Grandma Pat lets us have Cocoa Puffs.*

The same thing was true out in the world. As abusive as Grandma Pat had been at home, going all the way back to the 1950s she had always been a charming and respected pillar of the Ventura community. She'd been a travel agent and was quite successful at it, so almost everybody in town knew her and loved her. Years later, when her cancer finally came back and she passed away, the headline of her obituary was something like "Patricia Troxell Loved Everyone." I can see now how crazy-making all of that must have been for my mom, for her trauma and pain to never be seen or acknowledged.

> People inflict pain in order to share the pain that they're feeling inside.

My mother learned to abuse in order to show that she was abused. All of my mom's temper tantrums and her self-destructive behavior, all of it was an attempt to shout out to the world, "Don't you see? Don't you see how much pain I'm in? Don't you see what this horrible woman did to me?" But the world couldn't see it, so the world never acknowledged it, so my mom's abuse continued.

It not only continued, by the way; it escalated. Over time, always being right was no longer the ticket to being loved; always being right was the surefire way to drive off the people she needed to give her the love she so sorely lacked. Over time, my mother's ability to inflict pain on us diminished because we were developing our own unhealthy coping mechanisms to protect ourselves against her. Our synapses and neural pathways were frantically rewiring themselves, creating subconscious behaviors that would help us avoid trauma and seek out pleasure and love in our own dysfunctional, self-destructive ways. We stayed away from her; we threw ourselves into unhealthy relationships with other people and our different obsessions.

And so, over time, as my mother was less and less able to diffuse her pain by inflicting it on others, she turned more and more to dulling the pain inside herself.

When it came to self-medication, booze was always my mom's anesthetic of choice. She dabbled in pills over the years, but it was mostly booze. Same with Gary. By the time we were teenagers, they were both drinkers. They loved wine, but they would drink anything. In later years, as she continued to disintegrate, she started switching to much heavier stuff, typically vodka.

Her other escape was shopping. Practically her sole passion in life was going to all the department stores and hitting the clearance racks, chasing the little dopamine hits that came with finding a big sale or a hidden gem. She was always spending more money than we had. She'd go out and find some dress in a thrift store for ten dollars, talking about how it was such a great find because it would have been one hundred dollars at a high-end consignment shop. So in her mind it was like she was saving ninety dollars when really she was wasting ten dollars we couldn't afford to spend to begin with. It didn't make any sense, but it made sense to her. Even when she couldn't find a win anywhere else, she could get a win by going and finding a big sale on something and telling herself that she was being super savvy by outsmarting the system, playing it like a wardrobe stock market. That's where she found an identity.

The problem started during her first marriage, in the early eighties when regular families had easy access to credit cards for the first time. When that happened, my mom was like, "Oh, it's free money! I can spend whatever I want!" She ran up hundreds of thousands of dollars in debt, and this was in 1980s dollars. My dad nearly had to file for bankruptcy, cancel all the credit cards in her name, and keep taking all those remote assignments because it was the only way to pay off the bills, and to his credit, he did. He paid off every penny.

Then, as with everything else, as we got older, the crazy got worse. My mom was getting older and more out of touch with what was fashionable, so none of the "hidden gems" she bought were ever worth anything to anyone else. My sisters and I reached the age where we wanted to shop for ourselves, and she didn't have kids to buy clothes for. So she started to buy clothes for her friends' kids. Then she was buying baby clothes for people she knew who had babies. Then she started buying baby clothes for people she barely knew who didn't even have babies, friends of friends who'd gotten married but who weren't even pregnant, all as a way of rationalizing her addiction to spending money to get a little dopamine hit so she wouldn't feel miserable at the end of the day.

Of course, nobody had asked for any of this stuff, and many didn't need any of it, so her shopping problem gave way to a hoarding problem, particularly later in life. The reality was, the older my mom got, the more the clutter grew. Which is part of why being in that house was so anxiety inducing. Now, more and more, the inside of the house resembled the inside of my mom's mind, which was an unsettling place to be.

I never wanted to spend time at home anymore. Ever. By the end of our three years in the Northwest, I had made a few friends, the other outcasts like me, and I was always hanging out at their houses as late as I could, hoping their mothers would understand my situation and ask me to stay for dinner. I didn't want to be a burden on them, but I wanted so much to not have to go home. My biggest escape was in rollerblading. Which, okay, may seem kinda cheesy, but it had just become a big trend at the time. I got into that big-time, and that's where I made most of my fellow outcast friends. We weren't the skateboarders and we weren't the jocks; we were a bunch of nerds off rolling around on the ice skates of summertime. But I loved it, because now I was mobile. Now I could get away, and I did. Me and my buddies would go rollerblading and do rails and stairs and go to skate parks and do half-pipes, but more than anything we would just skate. We'd pick a point on the map and go. We used to skate so far away from home, miles and miles, sometimes into the next city over. If my mom had ever had any idea how far away from home I actually was, she would have gone ballistic. Which, again, is part of the reason why I always went as far away as I did.

The summer before my freshman year of high school, we left the Northwest and moved back to Ventura. Gary had a new job; he was transitioning out of architecture and doing more work in digital audio and had some new opportunity in that arena. Driving back down Interstate 5 to move home was and still is one of the happiest moments of my entire life. I was elated. I couldn't get out of Seattle fast enough. Gary and my sisters were in the minivan, and I was riding shotgun with my mom, who was driving this big old U-Haul we'd rented. It was a beautiful day, and as we crossed over from Oregon into Northern California, Fleetwood Mac's "Don't Stop" came on the radio. My mom reached over to the dial and *cranked* it. We were rockin' down the Five, singing at the top of our lungs, "Don't! Stop! Thinkin' about tomorrow!" It felt like all the gray, dismal depression of the Northwest was behind us and nothing but a bright, sunny future lay ahead.

Of course, that wasn't the case, especially not after we ended up moving into Grandma Pat's house. My mom wanted us to go to Buena High School, the same school she went to growing up, and Grandma Pat had started seeing this new guy named Bob and wanted to move in with him. So rather than her selling the old house, it was decided that we would move in—back into the house where my mother had been psychologically tortured. Given that my mother had never been to therapy to deal with all the issues brought on by that psychological torture, and given that we were now going to be financially beholden to the woman who'd done the psychological torturing, this was maybe not the brightest idea. Because that glass of water was still perched perilously close to the edge of the counter—and you can't start thinking about tomorrow when your mind is still shackled to the trauma of the past.

# SIX

# *Know Your Type*

Once I realized I was able to make people laugh, I was addicted to it. But I didn't understand why I was addicted to it. I didn't understand that I was trying to create joy and love in the world because I lived in a world seriously lacking in joy and love. I didn't understand that I was flocking to this thing because it gave me an identity and an outlet and the validation that I was so desperately seeking and needing.

· · ·

When you're lost in the depths of depression or spiraling out of control with anxiety, part of what makes you feel so hopeless and lost is the feeling I had in Austin, the sense that you're all alone and nobody could possibly understand your pain because nobody has ever suffered the way that you are suffering in that moment. But that isn't true. Not only are people across the world suffering in the same way you're suffering, people have suffered in the exact same way you're suffering since the dawn of civilization.

Life on earth today may look nothing like it did thousands of years ago. Mankind's technological advancements may have remade the planet in ways unimaginable to our ancestors. But the core of what it is to be human has, arguably, remained a constant. We can still look to ancient texts from all manner of different civilizations, and maybe not all of it is up to date, but many of the basic lessons of how our personalities work and how to be a good person and live a meaningful life still apply. It's merely the setting that's different. Seen in that context, the struggles we endure today are not some kind of unique torture being visited upon us because of our own failing. Quite the opposite. They're universal, timeless. The thing that you're wrestling with? Someone in ancient Sumer was wrestling with that exact same thing five thousand years ago. Which is comforting, or at least it should be, because it means you're not alone. It also means that, just maybe, somebody's already figured you out.

As I moved through my time in Connecticut and got over my initial frustrations with vomiting up my story over and over again, I did start to find concrete and tangible help. The life coach I met with was especially helpful. She was much more "You can do this!" and less "Tell me about your father," which I appreciated. She was the first person who gave me what I felt was an answer, a nugget of truth, an actionable piece of information that helped me understand and reframe my life. We were discussing my career as an actor and my habit of seeking external validation for my sense of self-worth, and to help me understand myself a bit better she gave me a few books, the most important of which were *The Wisdom of the Enneagram,* by Don Richard Riso and Russ Hudson, and *The Enneagram: A Christian Perspective,* by Richard Rohr and Andreas Ebert.

I had heard a bit about the Enneagram prior to my trip to Connecticut, but these books opened my mind to a new and helpful understanding of who I am. The simplest way to describe the Enneagram is as a kind of diagnostic personality test, sort of like if the Myers-Briggs test and the zodiac had a baby. It is both psychological and spiritual. According to these books I was given, it's this ancient thing whose roots can't be fully traced because it was handed down through an oral tradition by Christians, Muslims, Buddhists, and Jews for thousands of years. It was believed to be so accurate that it was almost like magic, and the people who were enlightened to it didn't want it in the hands of anyone who would abuse it, so it was kept secret.

The concept, as I've come to understand it, is that everyone is born with a unique essence that falls within nine different categories of personality, different archetypes of character. There's a test that you take. It's one hundred and forty-four questions where you have to choose from different this-or-that options, such as:

[  ]   I have tended to focus too much on myself.
[  ]   I have tended to focus too much on others.

Or:

[  ]   I have been a bit cynical and skeptical.
[  ]   I have been a bit mushy and sentimental.

Or:

[  ]   When I've had conflict with others, I've tended to withdraw.
[  ]   When I've had conflict with others, I've rarely backed down.

You answer all these questions and the test acts like a Harry Potter Sorting Hat, telling you which of the nine categories you belong to.

These categories are not hard and fast. The best way to describe them is to imagine a spectrum of light. You've got ultraviolet on one side and infrared on the other, but each hue of light transitions gradually into the next. Red becomes red-orange before it becomes orange. Each of the types has a number and a corresponding name explaining its nature, though the names vary based on which interpretation of the Enneagram you're looking at. As an example, if you're a type one, that means you're "The

Reformer." If you're a type two, you're "The Helper." And just like the red-orange color, you can be different percentages of each, part Reformer and part Helper. According to these authors' interpretations of the Enneagram, no matter what happens to you in your life, no matter what programming you get, good or bad, none of that changes your identifying essence. You were born with that. You can be different versions of it, you can be healthy or unhealthy, but you don't become something else.

Each of these archetypes has a primary role to play, a primary gift to bring to the world. Yet each one also has a corresponding challenge to overcome, a deep spiritual need that can only truly be filled or satisfied through becoming your highest self. This gift and this need are intertwined and complementary, two sides of the same coin, the yin and yang of each other. If you are a healthy and healed person, you're using your gift to make the world a better place. However, if you're not healthy and not healed, you're too often wasting that gift, indulging it in yourself in a futile attempt to satisfy this need, which only ends in tragedy. It's a spiritual dead end that will not only leave you unfulfilled but also leave the world a poorer place for being deprived of your gifts.

Ultimately, society cannot function if we're not using our gifts for the good of the whole. There's a reason we are all these different hues of this spectrum. We're all a part of the same light, but we each serve a different purpose. We're all interconnected and linked to each other. We balance each other. We need each other. There is no right way to be. Not everyone can be The Reformer; not everyone can be The Helper; we are all complementing one another to make a better world.

My life coach thought it would be helpful for me to understand my story and my personality through the context of the Enneagram, and she was right. It might not be the right diagnostic tool for everyone; there are countless other ways to define and categorize the different types of human personalities. But I found it incredibly helpful, and fascinating.

When you take the Enneagram test, it doesn't tell you exactly what number you are. It gives you an array of highest probabilities, but it still requires you to do the work to read through all of the chapters and see which one resonates with you. When you read the chapters about the personality types in the Enneagram, you tend to think that you could be several different types, because there's a great deal of overlap. But then you get to the one chapter that nails you, and you almost feel naked when you're reading it. It exposes you and all your tricks. That's how I felt when I sat down and read the chapter on type seven, The Enthusiast. It was like reading my mail, all of my mail: good mail, bad mail, all of it.

*Oh God*, I thought, *this is* me.

And it was. The primary role of The Enthusiast is to bring joy. That is their gift to bring to the world. But accompanying that is The Enthusiast's primary need: their shadow motivation. You see, the desire to bring joy is coupled with the need to avoid pain. That is the true definition of the archetype, and that fit me like a glove. I was drawn to the world of entertainment practically from the womb. As I had grown up with a single mom in Ventura, television was a huge part of my life. It was the babysitter, the constant companion. I probably learned most of what I knew about life— or what I thought life was supposed to be—from watching TV. It was my first exposure to families that were "healthy" or "normal." We never watched *Leave It to Beaver* or *Father Knows Best* or any of those shows, the ones with the archetypal happy suburban nuclear families. For us it was always TGIF: *Full House* or *Step by Step* or *Family Matters*, and to the extent that those families were a bit more dysfunctional than the Cleavers, they were always dysfunctional in a "Haha, let's all joke and laugh

I believe God has created all of us to be conduits of love, conduits of light, conduits of life. If we can get through our own traumas and our own pains and injuries and find healing in that, it allows us to become stronger, more efficacious conduits.

our way through it" type of way, which probably didn't help all that much if you really stop to think about it.

I can remember watching HBO with my sisters, and I'm talking about the OG HBO: the logo flying in and the whooshing lights swirling inside the "O" and that big theme song blaring out of the TV, "*Da-na-na, na-na, na-na-na-na!*" It was the best. We'd sit there, no grown-ups present, and watch whatever was on, anything and everything; I watched *The Terminator* on HBO when I was like four years old. My parents didn't know, or didn't care. They weren't around. As long as we were occupied and not burning the house down, hey, knock yourself out.

At that age I had no idea what being an actor was, or how a television show was made, but I can remember, very distinctly, at the age of four, becoming cognizant of the idea that I could intentionally make people laugh. I learned that I could mimic people's voices and personalities, and do weird, silly gags, and it would make people smile. I started learning dumb kid jokes and I would tell them all the time. Once I'd achieved the laugh, I knew that I'd accomplished something. Because a laughing person is a happy person. I had created joy where joy hadn't existed before, and that felt like a superpower—a superpower that gave me purpose in life.

I was the middle boy between two sisters. It was my mom; my two sisters; my two aunts; my cousin Nikki, who was like our third sister; and my grandma. I was floating in a sea of estrogen. Our family outings were going to JCPenney—or Nordstrom or Macy's or Marshalls, or all of them—and shopping. As the middle kid and the only boy, I was always fighting to have a voice and identity of my own and constantly creating worlds of my own imagination. The television and the video games I played through the television became the worlds that I lived in and loved. I wanted to emulate them and be a part of them.

When I was around six, I started becoming aware of how the whole mechanism of entertainment worked. That's a television, and those are actors, and the camera is here, and the set is over there, and so on. That's when it dawned on me, "Oh, okay, this thing where I create laughter and joy in people, I can do that as a *job*?" And that was it. Something inside me clicked, and from that point on there was no turning back. I loved people, loved making them happy, and I put all of my eggs in that basket.

When I moved to the Northwest, I spent so much time alone, but it wasn't really a problem of making new friends. I was actually good at making new friends. Unfortunately, I was also good at losing those new friends because I was too much for people. I was Entertainer Boy. I didn't know how to shut up. I had no off switch. I was always cuttin' it up and doing silly voices. I impersonated Urkel on a *regular* basis. "*Did I do that?*" I had the Urkel lunch box, my pants pulled up. *Family Matters*, bro. That was TGIF. That was everything.

I used to go to my sixth-grade teacher and ask if I could get up and do comedy sketches in front of the class, and not for any special occasion or anything; I just did them to do them. One time I did this parody of Guns N' Roses' "Welcome to the Jungle." I called it "Welcome to McDonald's." I swear to God, I got up in front of a roomful of kids—kids who already teased me and berated me relentlessly—and I sang, "Welcome to McDonald's, we've got fun and games / We've got lots of French fries, we've got lots of shakes / Oh McDonald's! Welcome to McDonald's!" I thought I was a genius. The whole time I was up there I was thinking, *This is great. Everybody's going to* love *this.* Then, when I finished the song, you could basically see a giant, life-sized cricket in the back holding up a big neon sign flashing: "*Awkward Silence.*" It was horrible, and also surely part of why I ended up with loogies on my backpack.

You'd think I would have learned something from that. I didn't. I kept doing it. I would do anything and everything that I thought might be funny or would get people to like me. Amazingly, my teachers kept letting me do it too. They weren't concerned with what was cool. Their attitude was, "Let's encourage this kid to be artistic!" But what they were really doing was letting me hang myself in front of a classroom full of my judgmental, cannibalistic peers.

Even when my desire to bring joy was malfunctioning, I didn't know how to turn it off. I just kept going until I found the right outlet: theater. I started to do a bit of it in middle school, but the real awakening came after we moved back down to California and I enrolled in Buena High.

My first day of high school, I showed up to campus without a clue of where to go or what to do. My mom and my stepdad were always so wrapped up in their own dramas that they weren't very good at the technicalities of parenting, and because of that, I missed out on every bit of freshman orientation. My mom literally dropped me off on the first day and said, "Bye!" I didn't know who any of my teachers were, didn't know where any of my classes were, didn't know where the cafeteria or the bathrooms were. I knew nothing and no one, not a soul, other than my older sister who didn't want to hang out with me. I was all by myself, this thirteen-year-old kid who hadn't hit puberty yet and who, at five feet four, was way smaller than everybody else in my class, a dwarf compared to the seniors. It was brutal. I give a lot of credit to the grace of God that I was able to make it through. That and the fact that, after what I'd been through in the Northwest, this place offered at least a slight glimmer of hope for a fresh start.

For about a month and a half, I spent every break and every lunch period walking around by myself. I'd have my backpack on and my hamburger and my Coke and my cookie, and I'd walk around eating by myself with no friends. Eventually, I found another kid who also didn't know anybody, and we sat together for lunch. Then we found a third kid who didn't know anybody, and now we had three. Then one day I saw a flyer up on the bulletin board that the theater department was auditioning for *Frankenstein*. Having done a few shows in middle school and loved them, this felt like it was meant to be. I auditioned, I got cast, and I never looked back.

Over the next four years, I did every possible show that could be done. I did the one-act festivals, the fall plays, the spring musicals. At Buena, we had the Big Theater and the Little Theater, and the Little Theater was where all the theater nerds hung out at breaks and at lunch. I had to tell my two buddies that I usually ate lunch with, "Hey, sorry, guys . . . I gotta go," and I started hanging in the Little Theater every single day. I was there before school. I was there during school. I was there after school. I had found my tribe. I could be as nerdy as I wanted to with this crew. We could rock out to *ABBA Gold* and play Magic: The Gathering. I could sing and dance and do silly voices, and while it annoyed the hell out of the seniors, who were like, "Who the fuck is this fourteen-year-old goofball?"—it was okay, because they still cared about me and I still cared about them.

By senior year, I basically had all the credits I needed to graduate, which meant I could have been done with school by lunch. Almost anyone in my position would have said, "You mean, I can get out of here and go do something else? Hell, yeah. Let's bounce." Mind you, I wasn't a huge fan of school, but I was a huge fan of socializing. I was a huge fan of community, and I for sure didn't want to go home and be in that chaos. So I stayed. I took on two periods of being a teacher's assistant so I could hang out. As soon as I did whatever clerical work the teachers needed me to do, which usually took about ten minutes tops, they'd let me fly. I'd walk around campus, pop into other people's classes, hang out, tell some jokes, maybe make 'em laugh. Teachers would be like, "Zac, what are you doing here? Again?"

"Just stoppin' by!" I'd say, grateful to them for putting up with me.

Always looking for a bigger stage, I started doing community theater up in in Ojai, a little town near Ventura, the summer after my freshman year of high school. Over the next few years there I got to play roles like Huck Finn in *Big River*, the Scarecrow in *The Wizard of Oz*, and Jesus in *Godspell*. Most actors don't get a big break working in small-town community theater, but Ojai was a teensy town that is incredibly well connected in Hollywood because a lot of big writers, directors, and actors have homes up there.

In February of 1999, I was eighteen years old and starring in a play up in Ojai called *Marvin's Room*. In community theater, every night you go out and thank the audience as they leave, and one night this woman came through the line. She was this tiny lady, all of four feet nothing. I shook her hand and she looked up at me and said, "You've got it, kid, and I want to help you."

It turned out that she'd been a manager in Hollywood for a long time. She saw my gift and wanted to help me share it. The next day she made some calls down to LA on my behalf, introducing me to another manager who introduced me to a casting agent, which then led to my being signed by Endeavor, one of the best agencies in Hollywood. For the next three years I was living at home, bussing tables and working at a car wash while commuting down to LA for auditions. Eventually, I booked a role in a TV movie and not long after that got cast in the pilot for a new sitcom, *Less Than Perfect*.

*Less Than Perfect* ran for four seasons on ABC and built the foundation of everything that came after. I was only twenty-one years old, and I'd gone from being the kid *raised by* TV to being the guy *on* TV, bringing laughter and smiles to countless faces. It was my dream coming true. But it held the potential to be my downfall. Because as The Enthusiast, in addition to this primary role of bringing joy, what I was *also* doing was avoiding pain, and I needed to stop avoiding pain.

Pain is necessary. It is your mind and your body telling you, "Hey! There's something happening to you that you need to deal with." I needed to experience my pain. I needed to digest it, metabolize it, and understand it. But I never did. I never stopped to let myself feel it. I was always under the impression that to let myself do that would be wallowing in misery and self-pity, which is always a potential danger. But there's also a healthy need to sit with your pain long enough to process it. Once you have, you can go, "Okay, I've mourned it. I've seen the way it's affecting me. I've learned the lessons I need to learn from it. I've made my peace with it, and now I can move on from it." But Enthusiasts have a hard time doing that. We're always racing to get ahead of the pain, and because we're so fucking good at creating joy, we always have the ability to stay one step ahead of it.

Until we don't.

When you're an Enthusiast and you are not in a good or healthy place, you don't merely avoid pain by spreading joy to others. You avoid pain by numbing it—and the best way to numb it is through the "fun" of gluttony. Gluttony is the result of Enthusiasts abusing and indulging their gifts in unhealthy ways. Enthusiasts are party people, literally. We will drink and smoke and party because we want to feel it all. We want the highest level of that intensity and that enthusiasm and the joy of the ever-growing, nonstop party in order to run away from the pain. And that, too, is me. My whole life I've always loved to host parties—dance parties especially. I love bringing people together. It's in my DNA.

Enthusiasts can also struggle with FOMO. I've always had a hard time when someone says, "Hey, we're doing a thing on Friday." I struggle to commit to that party because, for all I know, between now and Friday something else may come up, and it's going to be way cooler than whatever this thing is, and I don't want to put myself in the corner committing to what this is going to be and losing out. It's the same reason why I struggle so much at the ice cream shop. I have a hard time deciding which ice cream to pick, because if I choose one, I can't

> Trauma is an incredible thing. It's a powerful thing, and what's amazing is the way it can ingrain behaviors in you, unhealthy behaviors that can last your whole life, and you don't even recognize that they're there.

have the others. That has happened to me my entire life. I thought I was just getting overwhelmed with options, but the reality was that I wanted to experience *everything*.

All through my high school and community theater years, I wasn't exactly living on the straight and narrow. I'm not so sure you could say that the jocks partied harder than the theater nerds. The merriment we had probably put a lot of the football players to shame. It was not healthy. I was getting high with my buddies every day. We'd find each other every afternoon and say, "Who's got the weed?" And then one of us would get the weed and we'd go get lit. At the time, I thought I was just having fun; I didn't realize how much I was self-medicating to compensate for all the trauma I was experiencing at home.

You may be able to bring joy to others while self-medicating, but you may well be dulling your gifts, and potentially wasting them in self-indulgence. Focusing your gift on indulging yourself is, in the end, a masturbatory practice of ever-diminishing returns. Eventually the noise of the party will no longer drown out the pain. You don't ever get healthy, and the hole inside you never gets filled. That hole can only ever be filled by sharing your gifts with the world, fulfilling your purpose and becoming your higher self—a person who is in communion with your community, your Creator, and all of creation.

There's the old saying that "Your greatest strength is your greatest weakness." The dichotomy of bringing joy and avoiding pain fits that pretty well. But the Enneagram adds a layer of complexity that I think a lot of people miss. The armor we create for ourselves, the coping mechanism we use to protect ourselves, can be the very thing that's hurting us in the long run *even as* it's propping us up in the short run.

That's what had happened to me. Creating joy for others kept me afloat—it kept me *alive*. I wouldn't have survived without my ability to do that. At the same time, it was killing me because I was only avoiding the pain I needed to reckon with. For thirty-seven years, I'd told myself, "I got this. Yeah, I've had some hard shit happen to me, but I can throw a party and I can have fun and I can be happy and I can go use my skills as an actor to go entertain people and surround myself with the people I've made happy, and I can keep doing this forever." On the rare occasions that the pain and the trauma caught up to me, I got to be good at fixing myself up and moving on. Something would hit me, and mess me up, but I'd self-medicate with a little drugs, some booze, some girls. I'd do whatever it took to patch myself up, and soon I'd be back on my feet and on the move again, never looking back at that thing that had knocked me down. I would always tell myself, "I'm okay. I've gotten through it. I can just keep going. I don't need to look down. I'm good."

But I wasn't.

# SEVEN

# *Just Be*

Talk to anyone who's been through depression or some major mental illness, and one phrase you're likely to hear over and over again is "And that was the only thing that got me through it." It's what gets you out of bed in the morning. You're a farmer and you have to grow food for your community. You're a parent and you've got a kid who needs to get breakfast and get to school. We are all, in our own way, searching for that one thing.

. . .

Part of poor mental health is not loving yourself, not valuing yourself. We're all walking around this little blue dot floating in space, saying, "Who am I? What am I doing here? What are all of you doing here? What is the meaning of life?" That is the human condition. But any time you feel that your life has a purpose, you can feel that you're here for a reason, whatever that reason is. Believing that you are here for a reason is a way to feel valuable and therefore worthy of being loved, which can be the thing that carries you through any season of darkness. When I was going through the darkness of my marriage, my ex-wife's dog was often the only source of motivation for me to get out of bed. There was another life that I had to go attend to. I had a purpose, even if it was a small one. Otherwise I'd just lay there with my mind spinning around, going, "I made an irrevocable mistake. I fucked it all up. What's the point of even going on living?"

A lot of us find our purpose and we think that finding our purpose is the thing that gives us value. It's the answer to the Big Question. "Why was I put here? I was put here to do this thing." But I don't know that that's the case. I think that most enlightened people you meet will tell you that's not true. I think the "why" of existence is merely to be. Your value and your worth as a human being are not connected to anything that you do or accomplish in the material world. All that you have to do is be. Just be.

It would be better if we all let go of the notion that we need to have purpose to feel worthy of love. I think that we all have a difficult time truly accepting that we are exactly who we are meant to be and that we don't need to be doing anything else to earn or be worthy of that love. Even if you have no social connection to others and aren't capable of doing anything constructive at this exact moment, you still possess the infinite value of being a human soul in the universe. You're still worthy of receiving God's love. You *are* God's love. We are, all of us, extensions of the creator's life, light, and love. This I believe with all my heart.

In the Old Testament, Moses said to God, "What's your name?" and God said, "I am." I think that is one of the most profound passages ever written in any manuscript, whether you're a Christian, a Jew, a Muslim, or whatever. You have the entity that we call God not giving itself any proper name or noun. But rather, it declares that *it is.* This passage is saying *sooo* many things, but one of the most profound is that God is not attaching any value to some title that may define Him. God is declaring His infinite and all connecting presence. A presence that we are all extensions of. But we ignore that, and we all run around trying to find some purpose to give our lives meaning when in fact our lives have meaning simply because we have them.

My whole life, my feeling of purpose stemmed from my ability to entertain and create joy, which helped me keep the darkness at bay for a long time. My mother, on the other hand, struggled her entire life to find a feeling of purpose. Her mental illness was rooted in some combination of (a) genetic predisposition, and (b) trauma from the abuse she'd suffered growing up. But if any one thing exacerbated her condition of not loving herself the most over time, it was lacking a sense of purpose. In fact, her whole life might easily be summed up as a failed and increasingly desperate search for purpose.

When I started going down to LA for auditions after high school, I deliberately kept my mother out of it. I'd seen plenty of after-school specials and read horrible stories about stage moms and "momagers," and I knew that's who my mother would be if I ever really wanted or allowed her to take those reins. I don't think I could have fully articulated why I did it at the time. I did it instinctively; I just knew. Then one day, my stepfather sat me down for a strange but very telling conversation that crystallized all these half-formed thoughts I'd been thinking.

It was the middle of the afternoon, and my mom and Gary had been having yet another fight. It was every expletive in the book, plus the usual litany of threats, my mom belittling and infantilizing and emasculating Gary as always. They were in the kitchen. I was sitting in the living room, not twenty feet away, and their altercation was on full, glorious display. I had learned to tune them out by that point. "*Fuck you, motherfucker!*" "*You fucking worthless piece of shit!*" It had all become white noise. I had turned nineteen and was still living at home while commuting down to LA for auditions, and knowing I had one foot out the door made it that much easier to ignore them.

After the fight, my mom stormed out of the house, and a little while later, Gary wandered out of the kitchen, and asked me to come join him in the office area. We sat down, and he took a deep breath.

"Hey, uh . . . can we talk?" he said.

I wouldn't say it was strange for me and Gary to sit and have a heart-to-heart, but it certainly wasn't common. We weren't exactly Opie and Andy walkin' down to the fishin' hole. Still, that day

there was something about his affect, this air of defeat about him.
I could tell he wasn't coming to lecture me or come down on me.
He wasn't drunk or ranting. This was the middle of the day, and
he was completely sober. This was something else.

"Okay," I said, curious what he was about to lay on me. "What
is it?"

"Zac," he said, "I'm going to tell you something very, very important, and I need you to listen to me. Your mom is going to try
to take your power. She's not going to try to take your money.
She's going to try to take your power." I was confused as to what
he meant and where he was going, but then he looked me right in
the eyes and said, "You cannot let your mom steal your power. You
cannot do it." And the moment he said it, all of a sudden, I understood: *Oh, fuck. This is what she's done to you.*

That conversation was truly one of the most bizarre moments
of my life. Here was my stepdad telling me essentially that I
shouldn't trust my own mother. The woman he was still very much
married to. Not normal, by any stretch. I
think he sat me down for that talk because
he realized, quite perceptively, that I was
going to be my mom's next victim, even
more so than my sisters. That was in part,
perhaps, because I was a man. Not having
any real power or purpose of her own, she
felt like she needed to get that from the
men in her life. She had eaten my dad alive and she'd eaten my
stepdad alive, and so now she was going to eat me alive. That was
one reason. But it was also because out of three kids, I was the one
whose career held the most potential to give her the greatest
amount of power, and therefore the greatest level of validation,
and therefore the greatest amount of purpose, and *therefore* she
could finally be worthy of being *loved*.

The tragedy is that my mother had all these amazing qualities.
She had intelligence, charisma, and passion. But she didn't know

> There are a lot of things that we've taken for granted, including our own legitimate, inherent worth as people.

how to consistently wield them in any kind of positive or constructive way. Her big claim to fame was the time she'd worked as the assistant to ZZ Top's touring manager for a hot second, and because of that, she was a self-proclaimed authority on the entirety of the entertainment industry. But she never had anything like a career or work that she found meaningful. She would go and get hired to be a manager at a real estate office or at a restaurant, charming everyone with a glowing first impression. But then she'd start poisoning all those relationships. She'd start telling her bosses how to run their business, and they'd be like, "Um, Susy, thank you, but no thank you. This is our business. We're going to do what we're going to do." But my mom was often smarter than her bosses and could usually be right about these gripes, so she just couldn't let them go. Her attitude would be combative and arrogant, and she'd sow seeds of mistrust and division in the workplace. Eventually her employers would get tired of it and let her go. Then she'd come home yelling and bitching about how her managers and bosses were idiots.

My mom got herself fired from almost every job she ever took. She helped get my stepdad fired occasionally for similar reasons. Gary could be arrogant and unkind, no doubt, however he carried himself more professionally with work stuff. But my mom could and would get in his ear and get him more wound up and angry about the shit that might already be bothering him a bit at work. She'd amplify the frustration into anger, saying things like, "They don't deserve you, those assholes. You work so hard, and they don't pay you anything." Shit like that. So then, issues that Gary had at work which could've been handled more civilly and constructively, ended up having catastrophic conclusions because of the emotionally toxic dance between him and my mom. They both brought out the worst in each other. And very rarely the best.

I think my mom did find purpose in motherhood, at least for a while, which is why life was relatively okay in the beginning. During the salad days in Ventura, her life revolved around keeping her three children alive. That she could handle. We were babies. We didn't have complex emotional needs. We didn't have personalities. I think people like my mom ultimately want kids because they believe those kids are going to constantly love on them. But after a couple of years of cuddling, infants turn into toddlers, and toddlers can be selfish little shits, as we all know. My mom learned early on that if she made us feel bad enough, we'd come running back to her, going, "I'm sorry, Mommy. I love you, Mommy." That would fill up her love tank again, and, for someone with a borderline personality, it worked fairly well. But it only worked for so long. Then we grew up and became moody, prickly adolescents with complicated lives, and she didn't have the emotional maturity to navigate it.

In high school, any time my sisters or I had a problem that required parental help, my mom would ride in trying to be the hero, invariably making everything worse in the process. She had a scorched-earth approach to parenting. The summer I was playing Huck Finn in *Big River*, the musical adaptation of Mark Twain's *Huckleberry Finn*, the show did well, and the directors wanted to tour it to some other regional theaters around California. They raised a bunch of money from the parents of the kids involved to finance this tour, but then some kind of shady dealings went on and the families who'd invested started asking questions about what was going on with the money.

Most of them went about this in normal, rational ways, like calling an attorney or writing a letter asking for an accounting of the show's finances. Not my mom. Instead, one night when she picked me up from the show, as I climbed into the sliding door of the minivan, she leaned out of her window and started shouting at the directors. "You motherfuckers! You know what? You're liars! You're cheats! Everyone's going to know your lies, you fuckers!" Then, making sure everyone knew how much leverage she had, she played the ace in her deck: me. "And I'm not bringing him back! You hear me?! My kid, the star of your show, is not coming back!"

All the kids and parents stared at her, like, "What?! Whaddya mean you're not going to bring him back? He's *Huck.*"

My mom did this, repeatedly, over the course of the production. Many nights I'd come off stage riding high on cloud nine because I'd created so much joy with this fantastic show, and then my mom would pull up and start screaming and I'd want to fold myself in half and disappear.

My mom jumped on those occasions like she did because she wanted *something* to give her life purpose and meaning, instead of being aimless and jobless, which she was most of the time. But she'd only end up sabotaging things, so then she'd no doubt get pissed at herself because she knew she'd lost control. But she also knew that she could never be wrong. So then she'd turn on us and light us up because it was our fault we'd brought her into it and made her feel bad. "You see what you made me do?! How dare you embarrass me like that!" As time went on, we stopped telling my mom what was going on in our lives, which would then deprive her of any opportunity to have the purpose of being a mother, so then her feelings of hopelessness and despair would get worse and worse and she'd lash out more and more—and round and down the spiral she'd go.

The thing about my mother and my acting was that she was never that invested. She was so caught up in her own issues that everything I did she only half-noticed. She'd drive me to rehearsals, sometimes begrudgingly, and I'm sure she liked that I had a hobby. But she certainly wasn't going around saying, "Oh my gosh, you've got this gift! I believe in you! Let me go and help you figure out how to make this a career."

But now, all of a sudden, she had a son who wasn't doing community theater anymore but was on the verge of maybe becoming a Hollywood actor, with all the trimmings and trappings that come with that. That's power. That's a purpose. That's "love."

For any young actor, getting started in entertainment is a long and frustrating process. A lot of opportunities come up and then almost pan out and then . . . don't pan out. Since I was still living at home, I'd have to drive home to Ventura after a long, disappointing day and invariably I'd vent to my mom about my frustrations, because she was there and because a mother is someone who's supposed to counsel you and support you. But all she ever did was seize on my complaints to make it about her. She'd start getting volatile and aggressive about wanting to insert herself in my life and my career, saying things like, "Your agents and managers aren't doing anything for you. I should be your agent. I should be your manager."

"Look, I'm frustrated too," I'd say. "I wish more was going on, but you've never been a manager or an agent."

In typical Susy Pugh fashion, she'd go off on me. "Oh, you don't know what you're talking about, Zachary!" Which would be followed by the usual, "I worked for *ZZ Top*!" As if that qualified her to navigate my path through the film and television business twenty years later. I always said no, which drove her more crazy and more crazy and more crazy, because she was looking for her purpose and had always been looking for her purpose, and she still couldn't find it.

When the pilot for *Less Than Perfect* got picked up in 2002, I found my first real taste of success, and she wanted a piece of it. *Less Than Perfect* was a multicamera sitcom filmed in front of a live audience, and I wanted my friends and family, including my mom, to be able to come and enjoy the show whenever they wanted to. But I also knew what my mom was capable of. She was sneaky, crafty. I told her from day one, "I need you to stay in the audience." But no matter what, with no credentials, she would always find a way to finagle her way down to the floor. She'd turn up the charm with the security guys by using the whole "I'm Zac's mom" ploy. It was impressive, I gotta say. She was a master manipulator. I learned so much as an actor by watching my mom.

Sometimes, without my even knowing, she would get down onto the floor, go and find the writers and producers, and cozy up to them by telling "funny Zac stories," gossiping and sharing information she had absolutely no right to share, which is such a manipulative way to ingratiate yourself with people. One time, the day after a taping, I ran into one of the writers and he was laughing and shaking his head.

"Your mom," he said. "I mean, wow. She's got some stories."

"Oh, great," I said. "What did she tell you, that I wet the bed until I was in sixth grade?"

"Uh . . . actually, yeah. That's exactly what she told us."

"Fantastic."

I had to call her up and scream at her. "Mom, what are you *doing*? I am twenty-one years old. I am an adult. This is my first real gig, and you're telling my bosses how I wet the bed until I was in sixth grade? What is the point of you doing that?" But I knew what the point was: it was to get in on the power. It was because she was so lacking in her own self-worth that she had to come down out of the studio audience to try to attach herself to the career I'd built *specifically as a defense mechanism to avoid the pain she had inflicted on me.*

Barely two months into taping the show, both for betraying my trust at work and continuing to be abusive, I had to tell my mom that she couldn't come to the performances anymore. Of course, that just set her off. "You bastard! You don't love me!" Which wasn't true. I did love my mom. Very much. There was still that kid inside of me who, like every kid, wanted nothing more than to please his mom. Ever since the day I decided I was going to be a famous Hollywood actor, I had told her, "Mom, I'm going to buy you a house one day. I'm going to take care of you." And that's all I had ever wanted to do. But my mom couldn't just sit in the back seat and enjoy the ride. She had to keep trying to take the fucking wheel.

From that point on, with my mom banned from the set, the abuse was relegated to long distance. In what became a fairly regular pattern, I would be in my dressing room, about to go down to the studio for the live taping, and my mom would call. Since she was my mom, I wouldn't have it in me not to pick up. The conversation would usually start out civil, but then as soon as I brought up whatever was going on with my career, she'd find some reason to start berating me. "If you loved me, you'd make me your manager. If you loved me, you'd make me your agent."

"But Mom, you don't know the first thing about being a manager in Hollywood."

"How *dare* you! I worked for *ZZ Top!*"

It would only deteriorate from there, and I'd be in tears right before I had to go down and do my job of making people laugh.

Finally, in October of that first year, not long after my twenty-second birthday, I decided that I couldn't do it anymore. I knew that my relationship with my mother was detrimental to my health, to my career, to everything. So one week when she called me, as the conversation devolved into yet another round of vitriol and recrimination, I told her, calmly and clearly, "Mom, I will not be spoken to like this anymore, so if you call me, know that I will get off the phone if you start speaking to me like this." Which only made her lose it even more, and as she started screaming and berating me, I said, "I love you, Mom. Goodbye."

And I hung up the phone. And in that moment, I felt some of my power coming back.

For the next few weeks, it was radio silence, with my mom digging in to prove her point. She was expecting me to cave and come back saying, "I love you, Mommy. I'm sorry, Mommy. Please forgive me, Mommy," like I did when I was a kid. But I wasn't a kid anymore. I was an adult, and I had learned my mom's tricks well. And, honestly, because my mom gave me very little in the way of actual healthy parenting past the age of ten, I wasn't missing anything by not talking to her, which drove her even more insane.

That phone call was the first tentative step in what would become a near-total estrangement from my mom. It was also the beginning of my sisters and my stepfather and other relatives always calling me up and telling me, "C'mon, Zac. You can't not talk to her. She's your mom! You gotta call her."

"I know she's my mom," I'd say, "and I love my mom, but this is unbelievably unhealthy, and I will not devalue myself by putting up with it."

All of my friends were telling me, "You're absolutely doing the right thing." Inside my family, however, everyone was still beholden to that deeply ingrained, learned behavior, that we were all supposed to twist and contort our lives to pacify her. But I stood my ground.

That first year on *Less Than Perfect*, Thanksgiving was fast approaching, and the radio silence continued. I wanted to go home because I wanted to see the rest of my family, but I also knew there would be some kind of drama waiting for me and, sure enough, there was.

As my mom went through life, burning bridge after bridge after bridge, one of her go-to moves was always to turn to someone totally out of the loop of whatever the latest crisis was, who had no context whatsoever, like her new friend Janet at work. She'd go to Janet with her big sob story about how nobody loved her and everybody was mistreating her, and then Janet would say, "Oh my *God*, Susy. I am *so* sorry, and that's *so* unfair, and I can't *believe* they would do that." This would generate the feedback loop of sympathy my mom felt she deserved. Then, armed with Janet's opinion, she'd come back and throw it in your face. "Well, *Janet* thinks you're being absolutely *horrible* to me." Happened over and over. It was textbook.

Adam was a family friend who's about ten years older than me. My mom had—briefly, before getting herself fired—managed a restaurant when we lived up in Olympia, and Adam was this good-natured dude who'd worked with her as a server before moving to Idaho to become a chef and, apparently, some kind of expert mushroom forager. We'd all kept in touch over the years. A few days before Thanksgiving, Gary called and told me that Adam was coming in and asked if I could pick him up at the airport and let him stay with me for a couple days before we drove up to Ventura. I was happy to do it, so I picked up Adam at LAX and over the next couple of days he hung out with me at *Less Than Perfect,* enjoying the whole behind-the-scenes Hollywood experience. Then one night, we were out on my back patio having a cigarette and he said, "Zac, I don't get it."

"You don't get what?"

"Your mom, for like the last month, has been calling me in tears, talking about how bad of a son you've been, about how Hollywood's 'changed' you, and I gotta be honest, I don't see it. I don't understand what's going on."

I kind of chuckled a bit. "Adam, you have no idea what you're dealing with," I said. "I know you think that you know my mom, and you certainly do know my mom from back in the day, but you don't know my mom nearly as well as you think you do, and you don't know who she is now, for sure." I then tried to explain all the destructive ways that my mother had been trying to insert herself into my life and my career and how I'd had to put a stop it.

"Well," he said, "we should all sit down and talk about this."

"Oh, no, no, no, no," I said. "You don't understand. There is no way you're going to have a rational conversation with my mom. She won't bend. She won't budge. She doesn't apologize. This isn't about getting to the truth. Because there is no truth outside of my mom's truth. If you cross her, if you disagree with her, if you so much as say, 'Well, Susy, maybe Zac has a point . . .' she will turn on you, on a dime, and eviscerate you in front of God and everybody. You don't understand her."

"No, no, no, no, Zac. I know your mom. We gotta do it."

"Dude, it's not going to happen. I'm not going to do it. It's not a good idea. For any of us."

Fast-forward to Thanksgiving. We drove up to Ventura. Dinner itself was reasonably awkward, but we got through it. I left Adam at my parents' and managed to slip out without incident, and I stayed at my sister's that night. The next day, I realized I'd forgotten something at my parents' house, and I drove over to grab it. When I walked in the door, my mom and Gary and Adam were all standing there, almost as if they'd been waiting for me, like an intervention.

"We need to talk," Gary said.

"Uh . . . no, we don't," I said.

I stood there, staring at all of them like they were crazy, but especially at Gary, because I knew *he* knew this was crazy because of the whole heart-to-heart about not letting my mother take my power. But Gary was a broken man. Gary was also an abuser in his own right, so here we were.

"We are not going to talk," I said. "I'm happy to talk when it is the right time to talk, with a therapist or a counselor, but I won't do it now."

"No, Zac, we're doing this."

"Gary. Mom. Adam. I'm not going to do this. I'm telling you, I promise you, this is not a good idea."

"Zac, we're doing it."

Finally, realizing I wasn't getting out of that house without a confrontation, I threw up my hands. "Okay," I said. "I warned you. Let it be on the record I've said this is not going to end well. Let's go."

My mom immediately launched into this tirade. The whole thing was kind of all over the place, to be honest, full of cruel, petty snipes, variations on the same horrible things she'd been saying for months. I don't recall many of the details, because the whole conversation is overshadowed in my memory by the way that it ended. What I recall is that, at one point, my mom said something that was totally out of line, something nasty about me. Hearing my mom say this horrible thing, Adam turned to her and said, "Now Susy, that doesn't seem fair."

Up until to that point, in my mom's mind, this little showdown of hers was three against one. She thought Adam was her ringer; she'd primed him and groomed him with her sob stories. But the second he ventured out in defense of me, she turned on him, whiplash fast, and said, "I *never* liked you. I *never* trusted you. You're a *wolf* in sheep's clothing!"

It was just like I'd told him: on a dime.

I looked at Adam and—almost like in a movie—his face went ashen white. From that point on, Adam was catatonic. He sat there in his chair, completely quiet. Now that she'd lost her accomplice, my mom retreated to her default modus operandi: being as hurtful as possible. "I'm going to lay waste to this kid. I'm going to put some pain in him, so he feels like he's in the wrong and I am the victim." As she was saying all this shit that was completely out of line and untrue, I stepped up to rebut her on it, and she snapped.

> If you respond to hate with hate, then hate wins. If you can temper your own ego when attacked, you can begin to see the fear and pain your attacker feels.

"You know what, Zachary?" she said. "I'd be happier today if you were *dead.*"

I have to say, I was a bit stunned. By that point in my life, there was little my mother could say or do that surprised me, but this was a new low even for her.

But the thing about my mom's tirades was that she was all bark and no bite, and I knew that. I knew she didn't actually want me dead. This was just her extremely unhealthy way of trying to get people to recognize her pain and cater to it. Still, this needed to stop.

My first instinct was to somehow document that this was happening. My mom was a queen of never admitting to something when she was called on it. My whole life, whenever she said horrible shit, you could quote it back to her verbatim two hours later, and she'd say, "I *never* said that." We all knew the tactic; it was part of the crazy-making, part of the gaslighting. Eventually, you'd be second-guessing yourself, like, "Wait, *did* she say it?" And she was always so overboard in her denial that eventually you'd say, "Fuck it, it's not even worth it. I'm not even going to deal. I'm not going down that road." So nobody could ever hold her accountable.

But that day, when she said she'd be happier if I were dead, I had the presence of mind to know that if I didn't get it on the record, she was going to say that it had never happened. If smartphones had existed then, I would have whipped one out and recorded her, but since I didn't have that, the next best thing was to have Gary and Adam as witnesses. So I looked at her and I said, "Mom, I want you to say that one more time, so we're all clear. I want you to say exactly what you just said."

She stopped cold. I could see the anger and fear in her eyes. She either had to acknowledge that what she said was out of line and apologize, *or* she had to repeat one of the most vile things that she's ever said to one of her own children and then actually try and stand by it. I could see her thinking, "Do I double down on this? Or do I admit that I was wrong?" Unfortunately, being wrong still equaled being unlovable in the twisted neural pathways of my mother's incredible brain. So, she took a deep breath, looked me dead in the eye, and said, "I'd be happier today if you were dead."

"Mom," I said, "I love you, but I will never be spoken to like that ever again. I'm going to go now. I want us to be good with each other, but it's going to require some serious therapy to get us there. From now on I will only speak to you in the presence of a professional who can help us. You guys pick the counselor. I'll pay for the counselor. I love you, and goodbye."

Then I stood up and walked out.

# EIGHT

# *Find the Patterns*

Without even knowing it, we can spend our whole lives stuck in feedback loops, repeating the same patterns of behavior over and over again, stuck in the same narrative we've told ourselves about ourselves. In many cases those patterns and narratives can be positive ones, but in cases where they're negative or self-destructive, we have to learn to recognize them in order to short-circuit them and reset them, like doing a hard reboot on your computer's operating system.

. . .

In addition to learning about the Enneagram from my life coach, another vitally important lesson from my time in Connecticut was learning about dialectic behavioral therapy, or DBT. It's a form of therapy that helps you understand the cause-and-effect mechanisms of the emotions and thought patterns that trigger certain unhealthy behaviors in your life. It helps you identify those thought patterns so you can see when you're getting caught in them in order to short-circuit them and correct them with healthier behaviors. It's very practical, almost like math. There are actual exercises and worksheets that you can do.

For example, whenever X happens, your anxiety starts spinning out of control and you start imagining all the worst-case scenarios of your life. Then you get wrapped up in those imagined realities and you start stressing yourself out over possibilities that don't even exist and will likely never happen. DBT steps in and says, "Okay, let's back up. Let's identify X. What is X? When you start to experience X, instead of going off in a death spiral of anxiety and stress, what's something you can do to help yourself feel better? A calming piece of music, maybe, or a breathing exercise." It's almost like in *Inception* where you have a totem that serves as your anchor to bring you back to reality where you feel safe and at home.

DBT is a way of acknowledging what has been said by many philosophers and psychologists for some time: You are not the voice in your head. You're the one who hears it. Because it's insane how our brains work, with all these synapses firing and different thoughts running through our minds all the time, some of them healthy, many of them not. Half the time you think something and go, "Where did that come from?" You are not controlling it, and you need to recognize, "What I'm currently thinking is not even close to real. It's not even something that I want to be real. It's my imagination running wild, and I've started manufacturing a false reality based on my imagination and not on true reality." It's about establishing a baseline of truth and then constantly reminding yourself of that baseline and bringing yourself back to it.

My dialectic behavioral therapist in Connecticut had a kind of East Coast New York vibe to her. She was a no-nonsense, cut-the-bullshit type of person. She was cool. She was one of my favorites. She was one of the people who I felt was more on my wavelength. I liked her approach to DBT because it was very direct. Like the life coaching, it was the opposite of the weepy, Kleenexy approach of psychotherapy.

To me, DBT was almost like a form of parenting, the way parents talk to a child—or, the way parents should talk to a child—when the child is freaking out about something that only exists in the child's mind, and the parent goes, "Whoa, whoa, whoa. Hey, hey, come sit down. Okay, let's walk through it. Calm down, calm down, calm down. Breathe. Okay. We're in a boat. I know you think we're going to sink, but look. The boat is sturdy. The captain knows what he's doing. We have life preservers and life rafts. We're going to be fine." You have to walk a child between what is real and what's fantasy because when we're kids our imaginations are big and out of control at times.

In my life, probably the most self-destructive feedback loop, the most debilitating inner narrative that I'd been living out, over and over again like my own personal *Groundhog Day*, was in my relationships with women. When I first arrived in Connecticut, I was still devastated about the woman I'd broken up with when I moved to Austin. The way I looked at it, I'd ruined my life by letting her go. Then, to help me understand how the end of that relationship was not the end of my world, but simply yet another iteration of a pattern, my DBT therapist took me back to the beginning of my relationship history and helped me break that pattern down.

I never had a lot of girlfriends in high school. If I did, it was mostly puppy-love crush-type situations and dumb, high school dating stuff. Then, the year after I graduated, I met Anne, my first real relationship. Anne was different from all the others. I *loved* this girl, or at least I thought I did. She was the first of an archetype that I would soon develop an unhealthy attraction to: Anne was essentially my mom. Isn't that fun?

Anne wasn't crazy like my mom, but she was strong and beautiful and charming and opinionated and judgmental and critical like my mom, which made her a representation of my mom and of my broken relationship with my mom, and therefore an opportunity to fix all that. Anne came from a good family. Their home was stable-ish and functional-ish. At a minimum, they weren't always getting drunk and shouting profanities at each other and storming out of the house, threatening to never come back, which to me felt like some kind of fantasy world. So naturally, I fell head over heels for her family too.

Of course I had no idea what real love was; most of us don't when we're younger. Being with someone feels good and so we assume this good feeling must be "love," so we chase after it, and I did. I jumped in headfirst and I gave that relationship everything I had. I was that guy showing up and surprising the girl with flowers and poems and all that hopeless-romantic kind of crap. It was all shit that I learned in the movies. I was Lloyd Dobler from *Say Anything*, standing outside the girl's window with Peter Gabriel blasting on the boom box. Only this wasn't the movies. This was real life, and those stunts aren't necessarily romantic in real life. Nobody wants the other person to give themselves over on day one. Nobody wants the other person to almost completely self-sacrifice right out of the gate—it's not attractive. We're not built to handle that other person's heart and responsibility like that. It's overwhelming.

Still, not knowing what I was doing, that's what I did.

Naturally, this did not end well. After Anne and I had been together for about four months, one night we were hanging out at her house. It was summer, she was getting ready to leave town to go to college, and I knew deep in my heart we'd be doing the long-distance thing, talking for hours on the phone late at night and all that. But that night, out of nowhere, she turned to me and said, "How do you feel about Candace?"

"Candace?" I asked. "Why?"

"I dunno. I just think you two would be great together."

I was gobsmacked. I stared at her, like, "Huh? But . . . but *we're* dating . . ."

In hindsight, I have to say it was kind of an astonishing move. I almost have to applaud her audacity. She didn't want to deal with me anymore because I was a complete emotional disaster, but she also didn't want the hassle of breaking up with someone who was a complete emotional disaster, so she tried to pawn me off on her friend *while we were still dating*. Obviously, that was the point at which anyone with an ounce of pride or self-worth would have broken up with her and walked out. But I didn't have any pride, and I didn't have any self-worth.

Anne went off to college, started seeing other guys, and kept me around as a kind of long-distance puppy dog she could use whenever she needed someone to dote on her. And since I was an eternally devoted, I'll-pick-up-the-phone-anytime-you-call-me kind of guy, I let her do it. Because in the end, it was all about me trying to find love and healing. I was this heartsick boy, lacking love at home, and I didn't love myself, so I was desperate to feel loved. It wasn't really about who Anne was. It was more about me trying to work out my un-acknowledged pain. I gave up entirely on valuing myself or my own time. I gave it all to her because I genuinely thought, *This is how you do it. This is how you show them that you love them.* Then we "took a break," which was really her dumping me, and she started seri-ously dating a guy and eventually they got married.

> Reprogramming years of incorrect teachings isn't an overnight task. Stay diligent. Trust the process. Know that your thoughts and feelings are temporal, and ultimately manageable.

When I got dumped by Anne, it *destroyed* me, and what started at that moment was this pattern of relationships that were always four months and out, four months and out, four months and out. I'd start dating a girl—always a girl who, looking back, I can now say was some version of my mother—and I would lose myself in this girl and her family. I'd be that guy showing up with the flowers and the chocolates, and it would scare them off and they'd be like, "Uh, yeah. We're just dating, so . . . " and then somewhere around the four-month mark, it would all fall apart.

Every time a relationship fell apart, it would destroy me, again. So I'd run right out and throw myself at the next girl, hoping to feel loved, hoping to feel worthy. No matter how bad the relation-ship was I'd cling to it for dear life because I was terrified of being heartbroken, which only guaranteed that soon, probably around four months or so, I would be heartbroken yet again.

Then I met the woman I was destined to marry.

(I don't know what the opposite of a spoiler alert is. "Unspoiler alert," perhaps? Regardless of what you'd call it, here's where I'll pause to say it: I'm not going to write a whole lot about my marriage in this book. As the internet will tell you, I was briefly and unsuccessfully married to someone a few years ago, but it simply wouldn't be fair to her to go into too much detail about things she has every right to keep private. So, consider yourself not spoiled. What I will write about, however, are the reasons why I rushed headlong into that ill-fated marriage and the consequences I endured as a result.)

When I say I met the woman I was "destined" to marry, I don't mean "destined" in any sort of magical, storybook-romance kind of way, although that is certainly how it felt at the time. With proper hindsight and therapy, when I say "destined," what I mean is that I had grown up in a dysfunctional home and was stuck in a repeating loop of unhealthy behavior and bad programming. Then I met someone who had also grown up in a dysfunctional home who was stuck in her own repeating loop of unhealthy behavior and bad programming. So when we met, it was practically preordained that we would bring all of our unhealthy behavior and bad programming to the table and make a dysfunctional home of our own.

And that's what we did.

It started out the way my relationships always had, with me throwing myself into the deep end face-first, only for some reason it was even more intense than ever before. Our first date was one of those magical nights where everything clicks and you stay up and hang out all night long, talking and talking and talking. From the jump we were both talking about what we wanted in life, how we were both Christian, how we wanted to get married young and start a family young. The whole night I was like, "Yes, yes, yes, yes, yes. Oh my gosh, I can't believe it. This girl is perfect, and she likes me. This is it. Good thing you didn't end up with anybody else, Zac, because she's the one."

We lived in separate cities. Different countries, even. I was film-ing *Less Than Perfect* in LA and she was working in Vancouver, but despite the distance we talked on the phone every day, multiple times a day, and within a week and a half we were legitimately talking about getting married. Which was totally fine by me and *not abnormal at all.* Because of our different schedules, I had a lot more free time. And because I was the hopeless romantic, I started flying up to Vancouver to hang out with her whenever I could.

One week we took a road trip through the Canadian Rockies, which are gorgeous, by the way. We were both into the band Weezer at the time, especially this one song, "Only in Dreams," the last track from their Blue Album. At that age, loving the same band is one of those silly things we attribute to being an important marker of compatibility or like-mindedness. We played "Only in Dreams" over and over again the whole trip, and she had this funny, quirky thing where she would always to drum out the beats with her fingers and get into the music. She was everything I thought I ever wanted. I was a goner. I was all in.

I was also psyched by the idea of marrying young, which was certainly not the norm for a twenty-three-year-old guy in LA at the time. Everyone my age wanted to be out in the bars, single, having a ball. Not me. I wanted a family.

Even aside from subconsciously wanting to fix all the problems of my own family—which I obviously did—I wanted to be a young dad, a fantasy I had that was driven by this one particularly vivid memory of playing catch with my dad. I was ten and he was forty-four, but he was an old forty-four; he's never taken care of himself. Sometimes I'd throw the ball and it would get by him, and he'd have to slowly turn around and trudge over and bend down to pick up the ball, and it would take forever. Then he'd get the ball and come trudging back over and throw it to me. Never did he complain, but I always felt like I was making this a difficult thing for him that he wasn't enjoying. I didn't ever want to be like that for my kids. Whenever I imagined playing catch, I wanted to be out there in the yard, killing it like Ozzie Smith. Now I saw that dream coming true.

It just felt right. Everything about it felt amazing. Of all the other girls I'd loved—or thought I'd loved given my understanding of love at the time—none of them had felt as perfect as this. She checked all the boxes, all the way down to silly things like loving the same deep cut from the same Weezer album. We were going to get married, have kids, do the whole deal. I was going to have a family, a functional one, a loving one—and then suddenly I wasn't.

That fall my birthday rolled around and she was supposed to come down for it but then she cancelled at the last minute, and from there the relationship started to crumble. Whenever we talked, she'd be crying and confused and, in my estimation, tap-dancing around wanting to break up but not having the courage to do it. So finally I said, "Okay, I'll say it if you can't. Let's take some time off. We'll break up, you go figure out what you need to figure out, and then you call me and let me know when you do."

She agreed and we hung up the phone and, in the moment, I was proud of myself. I was doing the mature thing, the not-totally-obsessed-lovesick-needy-guy thing. I was backing off and giving her the space that she needed. And because I was so supremely confident that she and I were destined to be together, for a few weeks I was totally fine. I thought, *We're both young. She'll take a few months, figure a few things out, and then she'll call me up and we'll live happily ever after.*

Then I never heard from her again. It was like she'd vanished off the face of the earth. For a couple of months, I was still in denial about it all. I played it cool, didn't go flying off to Canada to go flinging myself with flowers at her doorstep. But eventually I started getting word through the mutual-friend grapevine. "She's kind of moving on," I was told. "She's dating this other guy now. She seems happy."

And the moment I finally digested that fact, it *totally* destroyed me. I'd allowed my heart to soar to such great heights, and now I was plummeting down lower than I ever had before. It felt like a divorce. When it all fell apart and she didn't call or didn't text—no closure, nothing—I felt like I'd been left at the altar, emotionally. Every other breakup I'd ever endured, the ones I thought were so horrible at the time, were nothing compared to this. This was the first time I'd properly fallen off a cliff. This was the first time I felt anything close to the darkness I'd come to know so well later on.

This was clinical depression.

Some people gorge when they're depressed. Not me. I waste away. I couldn't eat. I couldn't sleep. Every morning I would wake up at six on the dot. No alarm necessary. It didn't matter if I went to bed at ten p.m. or three in the morning. I was up at six no matter what. I'd wake up and my eyes would flutter open, and as soon as they did it would dawn on me that I was in reality and she was gone. I'd curl up in bed, weeping and sobbing and praying that I could get back to sleep because my dreams were my only escape from my miserable reality.

Some mornings I would get up and try to go for a run, but pretty soon I would start breaking down again, weeping in the middle of the streets of Studio City. As it turns out, you can't run and cry at the same time. Shocking, right? It's a difficult thing to do, because you need a lot of breath when you're running. So when you're uncontrollably sobbing and weeping, it doesn't make for great cardio. I would get as far as I could and start crying, so then I'd start walking back, crying and crying and crying until I got back to the house, back to the reality where she was gone forever and it was all my fault. *I'd* broken up with *her*, because I was an idiot and I'd fucked it up somehow, again, like I always did.

> If we are to defeat the lies that depression and fear and anxiety whisper in our ears, we must do it through the simple act of loving ourselves, and others, in the face of those lies, which conspire to make us feel like we are failures.

In the moment, I projected it all onto her. My pain was all about her. The truth of the problem, and what I didn't know at the time, was that I didn't love myself. I had no ability to love myself. I'd outsourced my sense of self-worth to forces I didn't control: to my career, to my girlfriend. I was relying on that emotional scaffolding to hold me up because I had no internal structure of self-esteem and self-worth to help me stand on my own. So the moment that scaffolding was taken away, I collapsed.

I didn't attempt suicide, but that was the first time in my adult life I questioned whether I wanted to go on living. Work was definitely a saving grace in that it gave me something to do. But I wish I'd had someone, anyone, who could have said to me at that exact point in my life, "Zac, you need to go to therapy, and you need to go now. It's the only thing that will help you to process and understand all this pain." But I didn't. I didn't have the training that a process like DBT provides, which helps you understand your own heart or your own mind. I didn't even know who to talk to, who to go to for counsel or wisdom. Estranged from my mom, the only parental figures I had to turn to were my agent and my manager, and that's not their job. It felt horribly lonely.

The most hardcore phase of my depression lasted for at least two months, but even after the darkness lifted, I was a markedly different person. I was a shadow of the guy I'd been before. Even with all the trauma in my life—or, rather, because of all the trauma in my life—I had always been this silly, goofy, outgoing, happy-go-lucky, cuttin'-it-up kind of guy. A hopeless romantic. But now I was far more jaded and calloused when it came to matters of the heart. I didn't date anyone for close to a year and a half. I couldn't. I decided if I couldn't have the perfect wife and be the young Ozzie Smith dad out playing ball in the yard, I would focus on my career instead. Which I did. In terms of my identity and my self-worth, I put all my chips on work, and with everything else I was like, "Fuck it."

When I did get back out there on the dating scene, I wasn't looking for relationships, just a good time. The only way I had to process my pain was to become numb and angry. Up to that point, I hadn't had sex with many girls. My Christian upbringing had guided a lot of my approach to intimacy. Mostly through fear and shame, unfortunately. I'd tried to be good. I'd tried to love and be loyal. I'd tried to be an open, positive person, but it had all ended with my heart shattered in pieces. If I couldn't have love, I would substitute pleasure and make do. I would fuck the pain away, and I did.

I won't lie: it was kind of exciting at first. The Enthusiast in me loves gluttony, and I fell squarely into that trap. I was someone who never felt all that attractive, to be honest. Deep inside, I still felt like this gawky, nerdy teenager, and I still feel that way even now. But to the rest of the world I wasn't a gawky, nerdy teenager. I was an actor on television. I was living in this town filled with jaw-droppingly beautiful women. Now, suddenly, I met their standards and it made me feel good. Just like my mother went out and got her little dopamine hits from shopping, I was always out looking for a girl who thought I was attractive enough, or successful enough, to sleep with.

When you have no self-worth, that's an exhilarating feeling. When you get it, it's like a sugar rush. It picks you up fast but then it drops you down hard, so then you're right back out there chasing it again. It's the same as with drugs and alcohol, and too often I sought solace in those vices as well. I never abused drugs or became addicted to them or let them interfere with work, but there were certainly stretches where I was self-medicating with them in ways that were not healthy.

I lived that way for a long time, all through the rest of *Less Than Perfect* right up to the start of my next TV show, *Chuck*. If you have the means, that behavior can keep you propped up for quite a while—for years, in fact. But it ends up becoming this endless cycle because it's not giving you any actual nourishment, because you're not finding actual love. You're not capable of finding actual love, because you're not capable of receiving actual love, because you don't know how to love yourself to begin with. And the worst part is, this broken behavior is not just hurting *you*. I hurt a lot of girls' hearts in that stretch of my life. It wasn't something I was aware of then, but it's most certainly something I take responsibility for now. So, if you happen to be one of those girls, and you happen to be reading this right now, please know that I wish you would've met a healthier me back then, and I'm sorry that I didn't get my trauma dealt with before it may have hurt you too.

So that was my life for the better part of ten years. The few relationships I had never went the distance. Then, by January 2014, I had finished *Chuck* and was living in New York while starring in my first Broadway musical, *First Date*. One night, out of nowhere, I reconnected with the woman I was destined to marry—further fueling my conviction that our fate had been written in the stars. She was visiting a friend of a friend and we ended up chatting over FaceTime. Same as with the first night we spent together, we talked and talked and talked. At first, I was keeping it low-key and casual— avoiding any mention of the fact that our breakup had sent me into a years-long spiral of depression and self-loathing. But the longer we talked, laughing and joking and maybe even flirting a bit, I started to think, *Is this happening? Holy shit, are we doing this? You've waited ten years for this, Zac. C'mon, buddy. This is it. Don't fuck this up. Don't fuck this up.*

That FaceTime led to more FaceTime and then texting and calling, and suddenly we were talking every day. That was mid-January. By Valentine's Day I was sending her flowers and planning a visit to Toronto, where she was working. I flew up, and we had what felt like an amazing time. At the end of the weekend, she dropped me off at the airport, we kissed goodbye, and I practically floated into the terminal, thinking, *Thank God I waited. Thank God I didn't marry anybody else. Thank God I believed in us. This is perfect. This is it.* Then I was back in New York and we were talking every night and, within a few weeks, we were both saying things like, "Yeah, well, you know, when we get married . . ."

In hindsight, same as before, all the warning signs were there—big, flashing, neon-red warning signs, which I would have seen had I been healthy or self-aware enough to do so. We were in love with the idea of each other, but we didn't know each other. And we never once talked about our past breakup and what it had done to me, or to her. She never said, "Hey, can we talk about what happened between us all those years ago? Here's why I never called you." Because she didn't want to bring it up, and I didn't want to bring it up either. We didn't mention it for months, and even when it did come up, I quickly glossed over it. I didn't want to make her feel bad and jeopardize this good thing that we had going. When I lost her the first time, I felt like I'd lost everything: being loved, feeling worthy, having a family. Now I had it all back, and I was petrified of losing it again.

"She's the one I love," I said, over and over again, to myself and to anyone who would listen. "She's the one I've loved for ten years. I fucked it up once, but now she's come back and it's meant to be and it was always meant to be. This is destiny. This is God. This was God's plan all along." So thoroughly convinced was I that I told myself I would do anything to show this woman how much I loved her. I would do anything to make our relationship work, even if it meant silencing myself and my needs in order to keep her happy.

Part of the reason for that was the same as it had been in all my other relationships: I had no internal sense of self-worth. I had outsourced my value entirely to this other person, making me so terrified of losing them that I would endure anything and everything to hold on to the relationship. The other problem, and what I recognize in hindsight has always been a problem, is my thinking that I always have to choose perfectly, that there is always a correct solution and a correct answer—in this case, a right way to be married—and you have to find it, and if you don't find it, then you've failed, and if you've failed, then you're worthless and no one will ever love you. Because of my need to pacify my parents' unattainable expectations of me by being perfect, that thought has been wired in me since I was very, very little—and it's completely wrong. There is no perfect way to be. But I was obsessed with the idea, especially with regard to something like marriage. I couldn't just walk away from a bad relationship. I had to make it work, and if it didn't work, it was my fault that it didn't work.

And, as with any relationship, my future wife and I were both imperfect people. We both struggled with the bad programming that we'd learned as children. I think she, too, was driven by the need to achieve a certain kind of unattainable perfection. We were both preoccupied with having our lives just so. The difference between us, particularly during our relationship, was that when I failed to attain "perfection," I tended to lash out at myself. When she failed to attain "perfection," she tended to lash out at others.

One afternoon we were talking. I don't even remember what the conversation was about. All I remember is that suddenly, she turned on me and she snapped at me. It was the first time I ever felt her anger directed at me, and it came at me so fast it was like the lash of a whip. In the moment, I froze. I didn't know how to respond. I was scared to start an argument over it or stand up for myself, because I thought if I pushed back at all it might lead to a big fight and then she could decide to leave again. So I didn't say or do anything. I swallowed it. I held it in.

In hindsight, I can recognize that moment for what it was: it was my mother and the glass of water, a totally irrational lashing out over something totally inconsequential. That was the moment, honestly, when I should have said, "Okay, you know what? I'm not doing this anymore. I will not be spoken to like this. This is not healthy. I love you. I think you're amazing. Let me know if you ever want to work on these issues, and we'll figure it out from there." But I didn't. I lapsed right back into the bad programming of my youth. I'd spent my entire childhood walking on eggshells, trying to be perfect, trying to never knock over the glass of water in order to not provoke my mother's rage because I was a child who couldn't live without his mother. And I had learned that behavior so well that now, as a grown-ass man, I fell right back in line.

It was an unhealthy relationship, an unhealthy dynamic. I was crying all the time. In her anger, she triggered all of my worst behaviors, my avoidance and my anxiety and my depression. And for my part, in my fear, I led her to believe I was someone I was not. She sensed that I was someone who wasn't going to stand up to her, or disagree with her, because I would just lie down. Perhaps in her own brokenness, that's what she felt like she needed. And in my brokenness, I needed a woman who was powerful and dynamic and smart and charming and beautiful to finally love and accept me.

Up until the day we got married, for me it was nothing but emotional tap-dancing and white-knuckle anxiety, as I desperately tried to avoid knocking over any glasses of water that might provoke a fight that would end the relationship. Despite living with a steady, low-grade kind of anxiety my entire life, I had never had what you would call full-on, Tony Soprano–style panic attacks before I got engaged. Now I was having them frequently. I started waking up in the middle of the night, sweating through the sheets. I did that every single night for four months. At the time, I told myself it must be something wrong with my diet. I certainly wasn't acknowledging to myself that it was straight-up stress and nerves brought on by being in an unhealthy relationship.

One weekend I was with some friends at a kickball game out in Brooklyn. I'd heard thirdhand that somebody was talking to somebody about how they were concerned for me with this whole rush to get married. So I went on the offensive about it. I called all of my best friends and said, "I'm okay. I don't want you to be afraid for me," as if I had to defend the whole thing. Which nobody had asked me to do, by the way. I could tell some people on the phone were bewildered, like, "What? Why are you calling me with this?" With hindsight, I believe it was a subconscious thing, hoping people would say, "Hmm. What's going on here? Perhaps he doth protest too much." I think I was acting out because I wanted someone to stop me. What I needed was somebody to step in with a firm hand and say, "Stop. I don't care what you say. I don't care what you feel. This marriage is not going to happen. Maybe you'll get married someday, but you need to go and work some things out first, because this is not a healthy relationship." I needed someone to guide me. But at the same time, even as I was subconsciously screaming out for it, I wasn't letting anyone do it. Taking criticism is hard for anybody, and particularly for me because of the way that I learned that being wrong meant failure and that you're not loved. More than that, I had no parents or parental figures to help me.

If our engagement brought on panic attacks, the wedding itself brought me all the way to the brink. The morning of the ceremony I woke up already full of anxiety and doubt, only to then find that my soon-to-be-wife had bought me a wedding gift, a Breitling watch, one of the big, expensive silver ones. Inside the box with the watch was a note she'd written, saying the most kind and wonderful things about me, and it concluded with, "I love you so much. I can't wait to spend the rest of my life with you, my Quiet Warrior."

In that moment, I knew I was doomed. I sat there looking at this note, thinking, *But I'm not quiet. I'm outgoing and gregarious and loud and silly. And the fact that she thinks that I'm this quiet, say-nothing guy is because I've been silent this entire relationship, and now I'm signing up to be that for the rest of my life. What have I done to myself?*

After reading that note, I crumpled onto the floor of my hotel room, curled up in the fetal position, and started sobbing uncontrollably. Eventually, I somehow pulled myself together to be happy-go-lucky Zac for the ceremony, and we flew to Bora Bora for our honeymoon. With all the stress leading up to the wedding, I had allowed myself to live with the delusion that things would be better once we got married, in large part because that's what she would tell me every time I was able to voice any of my concerns. But things were not better once we got married. Not at all.

I don't know that I had ever felt more alone than I did on that honeymoon. It felt like I had signed my own death sentence. If we were now married, and things hadn't changed, and this was till death do us part, then that meant I was stuck.

There was a moment after one of our many fights when she went out for a walk and I was left alone, sitting on the couch of our beautiful cabana. Looking out at the gorgeous Pacific blue, I thought, "I'd be better off if I drowned myself in the ocean right now, because I don't know how I can survive being stuck in this marriage." I thought about jumping off the back deck and sucking in a bunch of water and drifting away. Because I was convinced there was no way to communicate to her how much I was hurting without pissing her off, which would only lead to more pain. That seemed like a death spiral from which there was no escape except divorce, which I was terrified of because it would have been a public admission of my incredible failures as a person, not to mention a waste of everyone's money and time. It also would have been, given my spiritual understandings at the time, a complete failure before God.

Sit in the empty. Search your heart for what led you there, and trust that you are stronger than it.

The marriage itself lasted less than a year. We lived in Toronto for a while and then moved back to LA. Every time we were in public we put up the façade that we were "great" and everything was "great," and isn't life "great"? Then we'd be alone and we'd be fighting and miserable. I didn't know what reality was anymore. We tried couples' therapy. Even agreeing to try it seemed like a huge leap forward, but it was too little too late.

In early December we decided to separate. We spent all of Christmas and New Year's wrestling with whether or not we could still make things work, but it was pretty clear the end was inevitable. After the holidays, I flew off to Toronto, of all places, to film a new show, and I'd barely been there a day when I got an email from her saying that she was filing for divorce. I wrote her back in tears, saying, "I'm sorry, I'm sorry, I'm sorry. I love you, and I hope you find somebody who loves you as much as I do, because I really, really do." And I did. And I do. I still love her as a person and want nothing but the best for her and her family. But loving her was never my problem. The problem was I didn't love myself, and so I put myself in a position where I had hurried into a relationship that wasn't healthy for either of us. If I had loved myself more, I could have loved her from afar as her friend. Unfortunately, I didn't know any better at the time.

I hated myself for putting myself in that type of relationship. I already struggled with loving myself. Some days I even struggled with liking myself. I judged myself harshly all the time. My self-talk was horrible. As someone who took great pride in looking at all the variables and preparing himself ahead of time and not falling into traps and not being duped, I had done this all to myself.

I had to shoot thirteen episodes of this show up in Toronto and that kept me there for about seven months. Now, I was stuck in this city that I only knew because of her. The only restaurants I knew were the ones that we went to. Everywhere I looked, there she was. It was the dead of winter, and all I could do was stumble through the week, crippled by the shame of having failed and my fear of the judgment I felt coming from everyone as word spread of the divorce. Because I thought, again, that I had screwed it up. I had the perfect girlfriend, and then I lost her. Then I had the perfect wife, and now she was gone. I was too much, and at the same time I wasn't enough.

The thoughts of suicide that had first surfaced in Bora Bora now came back, but this time with a vengeance. Instead of merely wishing I could die, I started thinking about how I could do it. I was visualizing it, playing it out in my head. The apartment I was staying in was on the thirteenth floor, and one night I walked out on that balcony and stood there, looking straight down and asking myself, *If I jumped, would I die, or would I live and be fucked up for the rest of my life?* I couldn't handle the thought of jumping and surviving just to live through the failure and no doubt lifelong pain that would come with it, so I went back in and walked straight to the knife block in the kitchen. I was sobbing so hard I could barely see, but I pulled out one of the knives and I put it up to my wrist. I was looking at my tendons, thinking, *Wait, how do you do this again? Is it crossways or longways?* Again, I felt like such a failure that my biggest fear wasn't dying, it was the idea that I might botch the job, slit my wrists wrong and end up horribly maimed for life and, even worse, embarrassed. I took a deep breath, put the knife back down, and called a friend.

## SELF-TALK

The biggest lesson for me through DBT was understanding how horrible my self-talk was and how that grew out of my inability to love myself. In one of our first sessions, my DBT therapist asked me, "When you screw up, or think that you've screwed up, how do you talk to yourself?"

"I tear myself apart."

"If somebody else in your life, like your sister, if she screwed up, would you tear her apart like that?"

"No, of course not."

"Why?"

"Well, because she's my sister. I love her."

"So, why do you do it to yourself?"

And I was like, "Whoa, whoa, whoa . . . Oh my God. You're right."

In that moment, something clicked. And it wasn't like this was the first time someone had talked to me about this. I'm sure that people had been telling me variations on the idea that I ought to be nice to myself since I watched *Sesame Street* as a kid. But it was the first time I actually *heard* what I was being told. Which is true of life in general. You can hear something over and over and over again for years and not have it sink in and apply itself, but then you'll hear it in some new context, or at a time when you're finally open to it, and then it'll suddenly snap into place. That's what happened to me.

I think part of the reason I was finally able to acknowledge it was because I understood why it was happening. You can't truly acknowledge something you're doing if you don't understand how or why you're doing it, because you can't or won't acknowledge the source of it. But what's true is that we talk to ourselves in the same way that our parents talked to us. By and large, if your parents spoke kindly to you, if they were encouraging and supportive and effusive in their love for you, then that's the way you'll talk to yourself about yourself. My parents never consistently talked to me that way, and once I started to think about how my mom and my step-dad used to talk to me and how that made me feel, it started breaking my heart. I thought, *Oh my God, this is what I do. I've been shitting on myself my whole life. I have no patience for myself. I have no grace for myself. I have no forgiveness for myself. I bully myself all the time.* That kind of clicked for the first time when I was going through DBT. I realized that if you talk to yourself horribly like that, there's a good chance that you don't love yourself because you were not taught to love yourself. And, as much as I wish that all my impatience and judgment were reserved for just me, I've also come to the realization that when I was in my most unhealthy states, those toxic attributes could easily spill out onto those around me. Which is even more reason to practice radical love and acceptance with yourself.

# NINE

# Hit Bottom

One of the most gut-wrenching decisions you have to make about helping someone is knowing when to stop helping them. Letting someone you love hit bottom is a difficult thing to do. It's *rough*, because if you decide to let them go, there's always the risk you might lose them forever.

. . .

*itting bottom* is a phrase you hear a lot in addiction and recovery circles. To me, based on my own experience, hitting bottom means coming to the end of yourself, being truly humbled and on your knees. We all have tricks and tools and schemes that we use to navigate this world. Even as our problems mount and our circumstances deteriorate, we tell ourselves lies about how we're the ones doing the right thing, that we're playing the game and playing it well and all our problems are someone else's fault.

Hitting bottom is when all those tricks and tools and schemes have stopped working. Hitting bottom is when all the things you've used to prop yourself up in the past, whether it's drugs or sex or alcohol, simply don't do anything to erase the pain anymore. Hitting bottom is the moment when you can no longer lie to yourself, when the scales fall from your eyes and you have to confront the truth about who you are and the pain that you've caused, both to yourself and to others. Hitting bottom was the place I came to in Austin when, after thirty-seven years of self-medicating and white-knuckling my way through so many seasons of anxiety and depression, I finally had to admit to myself that I was wrong about so many things, and that I desperately needed help.

Many people have the presence of mind to seek or accept help well before they get anywhere near hitting bottom. I was not one of those people. Neither was my mom. For decades, she'd been navigating life, barely staying afloat with all her tricks and tools and schemes, drinking to dull the pain, hitting the clearance sales to get her little dopamine boosts. Ultimately, the thing that kept her from cratering completely was having enablers; family and friends who she could consistently depend on to either forgive or forget her transgressions, allowing her to never fully feel the consequences that should have come with her actions. Nobody had ever let her hit bottom. At a certain point helping becomes enabling, and we were already well past that point when my mom was caught committing federal mail tampering and identity theft to try to get out of a DUI arrest.

In the years after our Thanksgiving blowout I'd kept up a firm boundary between my mom and myself. For most of that time I managed to maintain a reasonably healthy relationship with Gary. Then, at a certain point, he started asking me for money, which I knew was going to happen because my mom was horrible with money. No matter how much Gary made, she would find a way to spend it all. I helped them out with some of the bills in months they were behind. I also gave them a car as soon as I could pay it off. I did it because I thought it was my responsibility, until I realized it wasn't. Children are not responsible for their parents. Yes, we should be there for our parents when they're elderly and infirm, but it's not our job to be there for our parents when our parents are acting like children and refusing to be responsible for themselves. Eventually, I wrote Gary back and made it clear that I couldn't give them any more money until we all went to counseling and my mom got help for her financial problems.

After that, Gary started drinking all of my mom's Kool-Aid and finally succumbed to her toxicity. They went to war against me. I would run into people, old family, friends, and neighbors in LA and back home in Ventura. They'd tell me they talked to my mom and were worried because she'd said the most horrible things about me. "Oh, that bastard Zac. He's all Hollywood now. He's forgotten his family." It destroyed me knowing they were saying all that to friends and neighbors I'd known my whole life. I just had to trust that people were smart enough to understand when they were being gaslit. Still, it was hard.

Then one day, out of the blue, I got an email from Gary. It was less an email and more a novella. If I'd printed it out it probably would have run about forty or fifty pages, single spaced, and it was essentially a manifesto about why I was a terrible son and not a good person. The first thing that struck me about it was that it had a preamble—like, an actual preamble that was labeled "Preamble." It was like reading the United States Constitution. Below that there was a table of contents and the document itself, which was broken down into sections: "Section One: Why You Are Not a Good Son." And below that, each section was broken down into subsections: Section 1.A and 1.B and 1.C. I have no idea how long it took him to write this thing, but it was amazing. And it was *nuts*.

I sat down and started reading. It was eloquently written and very intelligent, because Gary's an intelligent person. I read about half of it and then I couldn't get through anymore. Of the half that I read, it left me both laughing hysterically and sobbing uncontrollably because I couldn't believe that they could think this of me. So I didn't respond to it.

Then came the Dr. Phil and Oprah threats. They kept that up for a while. Ever since our big blowout, whenever my mom was trying to bait me into a fight, she'd leave me the nastiest voicemails, saying, "I'm going to expose you for the bastard son you are. I'm going to go on *Oprah*. I'm going to go on *Dr. Phil*. They would *love* this story." First of all, it was kind of laughable that they thought I was so famous that the queen of daytime television would just be sitting around, waiting to get her hands on a big Zachary Levi scoop. I was a TV actor on a show that was never a hit; I was not Brad Pitt. Still, in my twenty-seven-year-old mind, it was concerning enough. I was at peace with my decision to let my parents deal with their own financial situation, and I believed

> One can practice empathy without actually liking someone first. And through that practice grows understanding, and thus love.

that I was doing the right thing, but that didn't mean that I'd be given a fair shake in the court of public opinion. "Ungrateful Son Abandons Parents in Need" is a juicy headline, and tabloid shows like *TMZ* are always looking for some kind of garbage to dredge up on a slow news day.

I didn't see or speak to them for five years and made peace with the fact that they weren't going to be in my life. I never went out of my way to find out anything about them, but my sisters would pass me information here and there. There was never a whole lot to report because it was always the same old story: my mom's drinking and spending and hoarding, she and Gary fighting like cats and dogs and threatening to leave each other, which they never actually did. But the big story, which consumed the whole family and which I couldn't help hearing about, was my mom's DUI.

Apparently, one night she was out driving while intoxicated—which she did quite frequently—and she got pulled over. The cop approached her door and asked if she'd been drinking, the usual routine. My mom said no, which was a lie. Then the cop asked for her ID. Since she was driving on an expired license, she said she didn't have her wallet on her, which was also a lie.

So then the cop asked for her name. "If you don't have your ID on you, I at least need your name to run you through the system." At which point my mom, thinking she would just sweet-talk her way out of this and be on her way, proceeded to give the cop the name of her sister, my aunt Sally. Because my mom was a smart and wily person with a fantastic memory, she could recite all of Sally's information off the top of her head: address, phone number, birthday, everything. The cop ran the name, pulled my aunt's license up on his computer, and since my mom and her sister look similar enough, he bought it. Then he arrested her, brought her into the station, and booked her—as my aunt.

Gary then went down to the station to bail her out, and because Gary was the yin to my mom's yang in this toxic codependency, he didn't go to the officer on duty and say, "Listen, my wife made a mistake and gave you a false name. You have booked her as her sister. Her real name is Susy Pugh." That would have been the right thing to do and it would have saved everyone a great deal of drama. But no. He bailed her out under her sister's name and, in doing so, essentially corroborated that she was who she said she was.

Now sweet old Aunt Sally was going to be prosecuted for a DUI. So, in order to prevent Aunt Sally from finding out she was going to be prosecuted for a DUI, my mom started going by Sally's house every day to sit and wait for the mail to be dropped off. Then she'd rifle through and pull out any court notices or anything else that might tip her sister off, as if that were going to stop the wheels of the judicial system from turning slowly, inexorably forward.

Eventually, because my mom was also lazy, she got tired of waiting outside for the mail carrier every morning, so she had her sister's mail forwarded to her own house, where she could riffle through it at her leisure and then slide it back into her sister's mailbox later that afternoon. So now, on top of drunk driving and providing false identification to a police officer, my mom was also guilty of mail tampering, which is a federal crime. And it was all to no end, because my aunt started getting phone calls from lawyers who'd pulled her name and phone number out of the public records down at the courthouse.

"We'd like to represent you in your DUI case," they said.

"What DUI case?" she replied.

The thing about growing up an abusive household is that everyone's ego responds to that abuse in different ways. We all build up different strategies and defense mechanisms to protect ourselves. Though they had grown up in the same psychologically abusive household, Sally was nothing like my mom. She was the kindest and softest of all of the siblings. For years she'd worked as the receptionist at the main orthodontist in Ventura, the one all the kids went to for braces and retainers, and she knew all the families and all the parents. Everybody loved her. Where my mother had responded to Grandma Pat's abuse by learning it and inflicting that same abuse on others, Sally's response was to be eternally passive and kind. So when Sally discovered my mom's charade, she wasn't equipped to handle it. She didn't know how to offer firm, tough love. Her husband tended to avoid conflict as well. They had the opportunity to press charges and put my mom in jail, but they didn't. They let it slide. Even though my mom had been crazy and abusive most of their adult lives, Sally couldn't bear the thought of what pressing charges might do to my mom.

Absent my aunt's willingness to prosecute for the mail tampering and the impersonation, which were the more serious of the crimes, the police had no recourse but to give my mom a slap on the wrist for the DUI. She paid a fine and had her license suspended, and that was it. And, clearly, she didn't learn her lesson, because less than a year later she was picked up for a second DUI, this time as herself, driving on a suspended license.

Still, I kept telling myself, it was not my problem anymore.

Until it was.

One day out of the blue, I got a strange email from Gary. "Whatever your mother is saying is a lie," he wrote. "You can't believe her." Then he started rambling off all these strange requests, asking me to help coordinate getting him his clothes and belongings.

I didn't respond to him. I called up Shekinah. "Why am I getting emails from Gary like this?" I asked. She didn't know. My mom and Gary had threatened to leave each other so many times I don't think any of us believed it would ever happen. But it had. Gary had cracked. He'd had enough. I have no idea what the last straw was, and I don't care to know. I just couldn't believe, after all of the horrible shit he'd said about me, after writing me a forty-page manifesto about why I wasn't a good son, now he was the one leaving my mom high and dry, with no money and no roof over her head, and asking for my help in making his escape. It was crazy.

Over the next couple of days, friends of his started showing up at my house with armloads of his stuff to put in my garage. Over the weeks that followed, every few days there'd be a knock at the door. I'd open it, and there would be some middle-aged guy with random shit of Gary's, some boxes or an old computer monitor for me to hold on to. Then, the next day some other guy would come by to pick it up. It was odd. And then, one afternoon, I was sitting at my kitchen table when I heard yet another a knock. I got up, walked over, opened the door, and there, with a massive U-Haul truck parked on the street behind her, was my mom.

"I'm here for emotional and financial support," she said.

I stared at her, and she stared back at me. Then I took a deep breath, stepped aside, and said, "Ooookey dokey. Come on in."

It's hard to be mad at someone as nice as my Aunt Sally, but in that moment, I was definitely upset with her. I wished she had pressed charges against my mom. In fact, I had encouraged her to, because I wanted my mom to go to jail. I wanted her to hit bottom. With the crimes my mother had committed against Aunt Sally, I thought there was finally a chance to force my mother to look at herself in the mirror. Because I knew my mom. Getting a suspended driver's license was not the bottom she needed to hit. But being forced to sober up during a stint in federal prison, having been sent there by her own sister, that might have made a difference. It might have saved her life. But that didn't happen, and now here my mother was, darkening my door and forcing me to reckon with the same question Aunt Sally had faced: Was I going to help my mom, or force her to help herself?

I could have shut the door and sent her lumbering on her way in her U-Haul. Maybe I should have. But I didn't. I'd given up on having a relationship with her because she'd always refused to take accountability for any of her actions. But I thought, maybe, now that she was in my house asking me for financial and emotional support, I might have an opening to push her in the direction of making healthier choices instead of simply cutting her off. We sat down at the kitchen table for a talk. For a while she softened up to me because she knew she needed me as an ally against Gary, who was now the bigger enemy in her eyes. But the moment I pressed her on anything serious, it all went sideways.

"Mom," I said, "if you want my support, you're going to have to explain to me what's going on. You're going to have to reckon with why you are where you are right now. What has led up to this point? Like this whole situation with Sally and the DUI. Don't you think that what you did to Sally was wrong?"

And I swear to God, my mom looked me right in the eye and said, "I was trying to *protect* Sally."

I lost it. "Protect her?! From what?! From the fraud that you committed against her?!"

That was when I realized there was still no point in trying to reason with her. She had no remorse. She'd learned nothing. She'd rationalized everything. Less than an hour into trying to help my mom, and I was already done. There was no point in going down this road.

Fortunately, my mom wasn't asking to live with me, which I wouldn't have allowed her to do anyway. She had a friend, Joanne, who lived in a town called Santa Paula up near Ventura. Joanne was one of my mom's old hippie-Jesus friends from back in the day, and she agreed to let my mom stay with her for a while if I paid her some nominal rent. So that's what I did. I kept a roof over her head. That was as far as I was willing to go. I was ready to wash my hands of the whole thing once again.

Then, a few weeks later, the judgment for my mom's second DUI came down. She had a choice: she could spend thirty days in jail, or she could check herself into a court-mandated rehab facility. The facility where the state wanted to send her was pretty bare bones, the kind of place they send the real hard cases, the indigent and the homeless. My mom called me up, crying on the phone, begging. "Zac," she said, "they want to send me to this horrible place, but I know of this better place. It's up in Seattle. It's incredible. They're good people. It's a great facility. I gotta go there. I gotta go. It's what I need to get better."

I went online and looked up the facility. The place where the court was telling her to go cost a couple thousand dollars. The place that she wanted me to send her cost considerably more. Part of me resisted helping at all, as I wasn't convinced that she would take any of it seriously anyway, and therefore my help would still be that of an enabler. But this was also the first time my mother had ever even been open to the possibility of accepting professional help, so I felt like I should at least consider it.

"Let me call them," I told her. "I'll talk to them, and if they really are head and shoulders above what this other place is going to be, and if you're serious and this is going to help you, then we can talk about it."

I got on the phone with the woman at the facility my mom had been talking to, and within minutes I could tell that these people had already been twisted up the same way my mom twisted everyone up. "Yeah, we've been talking to your mom," the woman at the facility said. "And, oh my gosh, it's heartbreaking and tragic what she's been through and we want to help her . . ." And on and on and on, the same sob-story shit my mom had been peddling for thirty years.

"Oh, you guys have been so spun," I said. "This woman is spinning you. Do you deal with these types of personalities very often?"

"Oh, trust me. We deal with all kinds."

"No, no, no, no. Do you deal with master manipulators? Do you have people come through your facility who can gaslight you into believing what they want you to believe?"

"No, don't worry about that. We've handled everyone and we have policies in place for—"

"No," I said. "I need you to listen to me. I'm being serious. She will come up there and spin all of you around if you're not careful. She's a master manipulator. Please listen to me when I'm telling you this."

*If you can't control it, don't let it control you.*

But this woman kept insisting. "No, no, no, no. We've got it. We've got it."

Of course, they didn't have it, and neither did I. Because even as I was warning these people that my mother was spinning them, I was being spun myself. What I didn't know was that Gary had moved back up to Seattle and that my mom was trying to go back up there to find him and figure out what was going on with him.

Like I said, a master manipulator.

In my gut, I knew that the bare-bones facility was what my mother needed. Maybe that would have been hitting bottom. But I let my emotions get the better of me. I let myself get spun, by my mom and by people at the facility, who sold me on better doctors and first-class treatment, saying all the things they needed to say to get me to bite.

I called my mom and told her I would pay for the treatment, but I told her that the price tag came with an ultimatum. "This is it," I said. "This is the last stand. This is the Alamo. You either go up there and you do the work and you get healthy, or we are done. I will cut off my support for you. I will do it. Don't think I won't stop paying your rent. Because I will, and we'll be done."

"No, no, Zac, I'm gonna do the work. I'm gonna do the work. I promise."

So I wrote the check, and I sent my mom off to rehab.

Two days later I got a call. "Hiiii . . . Um, we're having a little trouble with your mom. She's very noncompliant. She taking over her group therapy classes and not letting the therapists talk and getting the rest of the group to conspire with her and turn on the therapists. It's been frustrating."

"Okay . . . And?"

"Well, it's unorthodox, and we don't know how to handle it."

"Well, what the fuck am I supposed to do about it? You're the professionals. I told you this was what you were going to get. You told me that you could handle it."

"Well, yeah, but . . ."

It went on like that for a month. My mom never turned it around. She even snuck off campus to get drunk, and I think she went looking to try to find Gary. Still, they didn't kick her out—I guess they wanted to keep the money—and she was able to do enough to stay out of trouble with the court and stay out of jail. But they sent her back with a report card, and the report card was not good. She hadn't done the work, and for me that was the last straw. I'd given her the ultimatum, and I'd meant it. I told Joanne that I would no longer be paying for my mother's rent and utilities. And you'd think that Joanne, being my mother's friend, would have let her stay for free. But she didn't. She said that if my mom couldn't pay her rent and utilities, she would kick her out of her home.

Naturally, everyone in the family looked to me to step back in and solve it, which made me furious. No one wanted to see her homeless, but no one else had the means or desire to help. My sisters, in fairness, didn't have any money to help her out. But all of my uncles and aunts could have helped financially, and none of them did. Any of them could have taken her in, or put her up in one of their multiple properties, but they didn't. And look, I don't blame them, because she was a nightmare to deal with on a regular basis. Everyone kept turning to me because I was her son, and I was making enough money. It was a full-court press. "Zac, it's on you. If you don't pay her rent, she's going to be homeless. You can't do it. You can't let her be homeless."

"No," I told them, "I'm sorry. I'm not going to help her, because I genuinely don't think this is actually helping her. For her own good, she needs to be cut off. If she's gotta hit bottom, then she's gotta hit bottom. If you don't want her to be homeless, you can step up and take her into your home or give money to Joanne or do whatever you want. But I will not do this anymore."

Of all of us, Shekinah had always been the closest to my mom and had always been the most like my mom. And just as Aunt Sally couldn't bear the thought of sending her sister to prison, Shekinah couldn't bear the thought of our mother being out on the streets. She sat me down on the couch one night and she begged me, sobbing hysterically, tears streaming down her face. "Please don't let Mom be on the street. Please don't do it. Please don't let Mom be homeless. I'll go take care of her. I'll drive up to her. I'll bring her food. I'll bring her medicine. I'll do whatever it takes."

Seeing Shekinah in so much pain wrecked me. I was fully prepared to take a hard line against my mom, but I wasn't prepared to do it to my sister, so I relented and I gave her the ultimatum instead.

"Fine, I'll pay her rent and utilities and living expenses," I said. "The bare necessities. But you're the one who's got to be responsible for her. You've got to handle her. You've got to be the one who takes care of things, who makes sure that she takes care of herself."

"I will," she said. "I promise I will. I promise, I promise, I promise."

So we moved my mom into a two-bedroom apartment in Santa Paula. I set up an account to auto-pay all her bills, gave Shekinah a stipend for everything else, and that was that. In hindsight, I still ask myself if I made a mistake. Should I have cut my mom off? Would that have helped her more in the long run? And the answer is that I'll never know. All I know is that in that moment I wanted to believe that my sister's love would be enough to save our mother's life.

It wasn't.

# TEN

# Check Your Ego

I believe that we as human beings are infinitely valuable, and entirely un-important. We are infinitely small specks of sand in an infinitely large mo-saic of infinitely small specks of sand. If you can grasp that, then your ego can let go of your pride, your hubris, and your fear. You will be ready to say, "It's not about me. The world's not about me. But my world is about me. I am about me, and I will love me."

· · ·

The ego is a fascinating thing, and it has one prime function: survival. It's tied directly to our sympathetic nervous system, which is what kicks on when we feel threatened; our modes of fight, flight, or freeze. Its goal is to protect you at all costs. It will do anything it has to do to get you safely into bed each night. A healthy ego, responding to everyday challenges, does so in a per-fectly normal way. You encounter a setback or challenge in life, and a mature ego helps you assert yourself calmly and confidently in order to solve the problem. But an immature ego falls back into the most extreme versions of survival. Every "threat" is met with a response similar to that of our most primitive selves. A simple daily challenge could be seen and felt like a lion stalking you on the savanna. Your ego kicks into fight-or-flight, and you do everything you can to avoid confronting the lion because the lion is going to eat you.

For a child, still developing and still unformed, an abusive mother is a lion on the savanna. Only you can't run away from her. She's your mother. So what your ego does is it creates all manner of defense mechanisms that allow you to evade and deflect and absorb the fear and the pain that you feel. I think of the ego as being like your armor, or an exoskeleton. It's shielding us. When trauma comes along and smacks you, your ego takes the blows. It may teach you to repress negative feelings and memories. It may teach you to take the anger you feel toward your abusive parent and displace it by bullying yourself or others. These coping mechanisms are unhealthy and bad, but our ego is doing them for the right reason: to protect us. In the short term, they help us. In the long run, not so much.

As my ego grew, it built up an elaborate system of defenses to protect me from the trauma I was suffering at home. It wrote scripts for me to follow every time I found myself in trouble. My ego taught me to self-medicate my pain with sex and drugs and alcohol, for example. But far and away, the single biggest defense mechanism my ego created for me was in my work. I found entertainment as a way of survival. As an adolescent, throwing myself into high school and community theater gave me a place where I felt safe and protected and appreciated. I could go out onstage every night and create joy in a hundred smiling faces. Then, after the curtain fell, I got to go out and party surrounded my friends who loved me and supported me. It was great. It protected me. It *worked*. Every time I felt pain, or was even afraid that I might feel pain, my body knew what to do: Get onstage. Create joy. Call a bunch of friends. Throw a party. Self-medicate. Rinse. Repeat.

I learned to follow that script to the letter. It became so ingrained in who I was that I forgot it was something I had learned—and could therefore unlearn. And you have to unlearn it at some point, because at some point it stops working. The ego, for all it does to protect you, can also be insanely crippling. Because every blow to your armor leaves a mark, a dent here and a crinkle there.

As the years pass, you're walking around thinking that you're still pretty smooth and intact, but you're not. You're relying more and more on this armor that's completely cracked and warped and misshapen. Inside of that armor, you're not standing tall and hale and healthy. You're all bent and warped and misshapen too.

The hard truth that I've learned is that your ego can only protect you for so long, and it can never actually heal you. Indeed, it becomes an impediment to the healing you need. The only way to get where you ultimately need to go is to not rely on your ego anymore. You have to shed your armor and stand naked and exposed and confront the pain and the trauma that you've been running from. Only then will you find healing and enlightenment and peace.

The stronger your ego is, the harder it is to let it go. I had, and still have, one hell of an ego. That fucker is strong. To endure all the childhood abuse that I did and still make it all the way to my late thirties without the slightest awareness of how damaged I was? That's some industrial-grade armor plating right there. But ultimately, in the end, it failed me, particularly when it came to the one area where it had given me the most support: my work.

Hollywood is not community theater, not by a long shot. The scripts that I learned to follow in my youth didn't necessarily translate when I moved from one to the other. Arriving in Los Angeles and seeing so much inefficiency and inhumanity on display, I couldn't believe the way that the system worked—or, rather, didn't work. Maybe it's because of the environment I was raised in, but ever since I was a kid, born with this particular head and this particular heart, I have been constantly driven to evaluate systems and institutions, to deconstruct them, to figure out what works and what doesn't and why it works or doesn't work. It's why I was so obsessed with that book, *The Way Things Work*, which broke down different machines to show how they functioned inside. Which can be maddening, to be honest, because you aren't satisfied a lot of the time with how and why things are done.

Because of my engineer's mind and my empathetic heart, I've always bucked when I feel like something is broken to the point where it's inhumane, or inefficient, which are often one and the same. The engineer in me associates inefficiency with inhumanity, because anything that's inefficient wastes people's time and energy, two of the most finite and precious resources we have in this world. Therefore, to waste someone's time, to *steal* someone's time, is also inhumane.

Words like *inhumane* may seem strong when talking about something like the business of Hollywood, but there are differing levels of inhumanity. The fact is that anything that treats people as a means to an end and not as an end in and of themselves is, to some degree or other, devaluing and dehumanizing to them. It is another form of abuse.

Because I felt so little love at home growing up, and because I had no love for myself, I'd found it in high school drama and in community theater. Those environments were genuinely supportive and rewarding. When you're a student, your education and development are the point of the whole endeavor. You are treated as the end and not merely as the means. In Hollywood, the opposite is true most of the time.

Being a professional actor is like being a door-to-door salesman, only instead of a vacuum cleaner, the product you're selling is yourself. Imagine going door to door and trying to convince every person you meet to like you, and 99 percent of the people say, "No, I don't like you." Now, put a rational, healthy person in that circumstance and they will understand that it isn't personal. The casting director who doesn't want to hire you, they're not trying to hurt you as a person. They're just trying to make their movie, and you're not right for the role. But good luck trying to convince a twenty-one-year-old man-child with massive mommy issues that it isn't personal.

The way the audition process works today is that everyone tapes themselves on their phones. But back in the day, what they'd do is they'd take a pack of hungry actors and they'd cram them into a waiting room. Then, one by one, they'd call you into a little sterile room and the camera would roll and they'd give you a nod and you'd "act." It was basically like somebody saying, "Dance, monkey!" and then yanking your chain and watching you dance.

For an actor, every time you go through one of these cold auditions, it's like jumping out of an airplane. It's that pit-of-your-stomach feeling you get with the tick-tick-tick-tick of the roller coaster that's about to go over the first big drop. You're standing up there, naked, and saying, "Judge me! Tell me if I'm good enough! Tell me if you like me!" For me, it's far more intense, far more nerve-racking than actually being on a film or TV set. And let's not forget that we're talking about *actors* here. Ours is an industry made up almost exclusively of people who for whatever reason need to go out and get emotional validation from strangers. Yet we've taken these extremely vulnerable people and put them

My mom was deceptive and manipulative, to the degree where it was insane to watch. She would charm people. As an actor, I was learning at the master's feet, because she was such a chameleon.

through a system designed to inflict the maximum amount of anxiety and abuse. When you start out, everyone tells you, "We think you're going to be the next Tom Hanks" and "We're going to make you a star" and blah blah blah. They'll sign you up on the off chance you might be valuable someday. If you are, great, and if not, whatever. Then they'll hand you off to some junior agent while they focus on their bigger talent, and all the while they're hunting for a younger, hotter monkey who'll be happy to replace you at a moment's notice.

That's often the way Hollywood works. You are almost always the means to another person's end. It's a system designed to separate the wheat from the chaff, and the "wheat" sometimes isn't the people who have the most talent. It's the people who have the most emotional capacity and wherewithal to survive the gauntlet of navigating the troubled waters of the entertainment industry.

Getting cast in *Less Than Perfect* when I was twenty-one was a godsend. I was now consistently working in Hollywood. No more need for bussing tables or washing cars. I was making good money, and because it was a comedy, I got to make people laugh on a regular basis. Most of those four years felt happy, but unbeknownst to me my unresolved trauma was still guiding my ego in unhealthy ways. Booze, cigarettes, and girls started to creep back into my life after I was pretty straight edge for a few years. Because twenty-one-year-old me was completely unaware that even landing your dream job of being on television doesn't actually substitute for true self-worth. But hey, I was having fun and bringing joy and had no elder to guide me, so my ego was having a blast.

But then fast-forward four years. I had lost the woman I thought was destined to be my wife, *Less Than Perfect* had ended, and as much as I wish that it would have been a platform to attract more work, the show didn't really do that for me. I found myself once again at sea in the endless door-to-door rejection that was the audition circuit. This would have been a great time for me to go to therapy. This would have been a great time for someone who loved me and knew more about mental health than I did to grab me by the scruff of the neck and throw me into a therapist's office and say, "I'm doing this for your own good." But unfortunately, I didn't have that person in my life. So: more self-medication, more anxiety, more depression.

> For the longest time, I couldn't see the wounds that my parents had inflicted on me. I couldn't see that my relationship to work was slowly killing me. I was blind to those things.

You might think that landing the lead role in a network television show, as I did with *Chuck*, would have mitigated all those recurring fears and anxieties. It didn't. *Chuck*, while never a huge hit, always had a dedicated and loyal fan base, which was wonderful. I loved that I got to bring people joy. The feedback I needed was never just the love from the fans. It wasn't just from the roar and the laughter of the crowd.

## FANS

The danger of externalizing one's self-worth is that you've given over control of how you feel about yourself to forces beyond your control. It's like pegging your emotions on the weather: it's hot or it's cold, it's rainy or it's dry, and your feelings fluctuate accordingly; you have no internal thermostat to maintain a constant temperature. It's an unhealthy behavior that can take on many forms.

A lot of actors find the love and admiration they need from their fans, from the roar of a crowd and the waves of laughter they get from a live audience. I do too. It feels good. But fans were never my drug of choice. The first people I would call Zac Levi "fans" were people I met after shows up in Ojai, kids and even adults who'd come to repeat showings of *Godspell* or *Big River*, people who saw talent in me and believed in me. When *Less Than Perfect* launched, we had people who loved the show so much they'd come to multiple tapings. This was in 2002, before social media blew up, but IMDb had these message boards where fans would gather to talk, and nobody from ABC or our show was going on and using them in any kind of official way. So I started going on, chatting with people, answering their questions, and that started an interesting back-and-forth cyber relationship with fans.

As the age of social media has ramped up and taken over, I still do the same. Like almost everyone, I struggle to have a healthy relationship with the online world and the compulsions it brings out in us. Luckily, however, I haven't become someone who's on Instagram every minute like a lab rat, clicking the lever to try to get a little pellet of attention to make me feel better. Which has been good for me, because fame is fickle. It will wax and wane, and at some point, it will go away forever, and if you're relying on it as an emotional crutch, you're in for a major letdown.

So despite all my insecurities, I've always felt like I managed to keep my relationship with the audience in perspective. One reason for that is because my relationship with an audience has always been more about giving joy than receiving it. I love to entertain, to give laughter to people. If they want to express their appreciation for my work in return, that's wonderful, but the truth is (a) my enjoyment was seeing their enjoyment, and (b) when you don't love yourself, being on the receiving end of someone's compliments can actually make you feel a hell of a lot worse, because you don't believe what they're telling you.

The real satisfaction I got from my work was when I'd get a call from my agent saying, "Hey, they're interested in you for this job." That would give me a big dopamine boost: *ping!* It meant that my hard work and my talent were being recognized. Then the call after that would be, "'Hey, they want you for this job." Another dopamine boost: *ping!* Then the call after that would be, "Hey, look at this great deal that they're offering you, which means they value you and we are good to go." *Ping! Ping!* Then the call after would be, "Hey, we've heard from set that you're crushing it and everyone's happy with your performance." *Ping! Ping! Ping! Ping! Ping!*

I loved that shit. I fed off it, because it was love from the decision-makers and authority figures in the industry. In other words: from the parents. I was still subconsciously looking for love and approval and protection from grown-ups, the same love and approval and protection I never really got from my parents. Receiving that approval at all those steps along the way meant that I was accomplishing what I had set out to do. And if I wasn't getting those signals of approval, then that meant I was screwing up somehow. I was failing.

Show business has always been a business. In any business the bottom line is the bottom line, and in Hollywood people have been exploited and chewed up and spit out for the sake of the bottom line since the days of the silver screen. But being on a network show at that point in time was precarious, as network television was starting to die on the vine. TiVo was allowing viewers to fast-forward right through the commercials that paid for everything, premium cable shows like *The Sopranos* and *Mad Men* were stealing the prestige and the eyeballs, reality TV was clogging up the airwaves at a tenth of the cost of scripted shows, and the streaming revolution was waiting just over the horizon, ready to clobber the medium with a final death blow.

The only way to squeeze more profit out of a scripted network show was to jam in more and more ads, to the point where shows were breaking for commercial so frequently they were less and less enjoyable to watch. Any and all aspirations about artistic quality had to be regularly hurled overboard in a frantic and futile effort to stay afloat. It was all about wringing every last drop of value out of this rapidly depreciating asset before it died for good. The bottom line was the only line that mattered anymore.

Because of that, *Chuck* was perhaps the most bittersweet experience of my life, one of the greatest blessings I've ever been given and also one of the most difficult trials I've ever endured. In the "count your blessings" column: I was the lead in a prime-time TV show. I was making good money. I got to work with an incredible cast and crew. They truly were like a surrogate family, and I love them like family to this day.

But the trials of *Chuck* were many. One was that the show was not a hit but it was also not *not* a hit. We always did just okay, and that meant we were always on the bubble. Every year, the executives at NBC would say, "Okay, *Chuck* is not performing the way we want it to. Tell Warner Brothers we don't know if we're bringing it back or not." Then they'd put a pin in us and go and develop all these other pilots for all these other shows that they hoped would be amazing enough to potentially replace us. Every year, miraculously, most of those wouldn't test well enough, and then they'd come back to Warner Brothers at the last minute and say, "Alright, we'll bring back *Chuck*, but we're going to pay less for it this time." So then Warner Brothers would come to the producers and say, "You've gotta cut your budget."

So every year our execution was stayed and every year we were forced to come back and do more and more with less and less. *Chuck* would have been a difficult show even in the best of circumstances. It was an hour-long, single-camera action dramedy with a ton of fight scenes, car chases, and explosions. Our first season, we averaged sixteen-hour days. If we ever got a fourteen-hour day we were thrilled—a fourteen-hour day was like a blessing from heaven—and we were shooting like that five days a week. But Fridays always bled into Saturday—which we called Fraturdays— and almost every Fraturday we were walking off the stage to go home around seven in the morning. And because Chuck Bartowski was in virtually every scene on the show, I got a day off once in the bluest of moons. To say it was detrimental to my overall well being would be a gross understatement.

I was losing my mind, but I was 100 percent committed to doing whatever it took for the show to succeed. For years, I told the producers and executives, "Whatever you need me to do. If it helps the show, I will go and do it." If they said, "Jump," I said, "How high?"

I did every marketing stunt they ever asked for. I turned myself into a human billboard for the show. At the same time, the show itself was becoming a sort of billboard for all manner of products inside the show. As each season passed and the tighter the budgets got, the more we came to rely on product placement inside the episodes. The product placement got so heavy-handed at times that *Chuck* became kind of infamous for it. The number of Subway sandwiches we highlighted in that show could have fed a small nation.

In one episode we were on a spy mission, staking out the bad guy's house in a Toyota van. One of the other characters asked what we were doing in this van, and my line was something like, "Well, my car is getting fixed, so Ellie and Devon lent me their van. Did you know it has nine-point surround-sound Dolby digital speakers and a full flat third row?" This was the dialogue we were being asked to perform in the middle of a dangerous spy mission. I don't blame the writers for these ridiculous moments, but I sure wish we hadn't had to do them. The truth is it was demoralizing. We weren't bringing the audience joy. We were selling them cars. It was no way to value people, no way to value the show, no way to value the audience. In the end, I would say that as the practice spread across network TV it was even bad for the bottom line, because it compromised the quality of the programming and only drove people to run to streaming and cable that much faster in search of something better to watch.

I would have done anything to make *Chuck* work. I would have driven Toyota minivans from coast to coast if I'd been asked and it would have actually helped. I was driven by my desire to bring joy to the fans who loved the show. I was driven by my love for my fellow cast and crew and my desire to protect them. But I was also being driven by my own insecurities, by my need to be perfect to avoid feeling like a failure, by my need for approval and acknowledgment from the decision-makers and my peers in the industry. Not only was I not getting it, I felt like I was getting the opposite of it.

In five years on *Chuck*, I gave every ounce of who I was to that show. I jumped through every hoop. On top of the eighty-hour weeks, I made every public appearance, tap-danced and schmoozed through every industry dinner, whatever I needed to do to help

the show survive. They took every ounce that I gave them. But if I
went back and asked for any kind of consideration in return—say
a lighter shooting schedule, or a raise—the studio head at the
time told me flat out, "You know, you're lucky to have a job." He
told me, in essence, that ultimately I wasn't worth very much to
them, and because deep down I already believed I was worthless,
it was a debilitating cycle in which to be stuck. It was terrible for
my physical, emotional, and mental health. And because I didn't
understand my true motivations for doing it—in other words, that
I was looking for love and approval from people who would never
give it to me to try to fill this bottomless well of need inside of

> By this point in human
> history and modern
> society we have
> constructed such a
> massive system of
> pressure that comes
> at us from all sides.

myself—I just kept doing it, even though
it was slowly killing me. I'd fought so hard
to escape my mom and put up boundaries
between myself and my mom. And now:
I'd gone to work for my mom.

By any objective standard of "success" I
had done well. Anyone who looked at me
would have seen a TV star with fame and
money. But given the nature of my job,

being beholden to parental surrogates and authority figures who
could seemingly never be pleased, what looked to the whole world
like a "successful" acting job was in fact pouring salt in the wounds
I'd endured all through my childhood. I had invested my entire
sense of self-worth in a system that is not geared at all to care about
my actual well-being as a person.

And yet: I never broke down. Never once in those five years
did I experience the kind of mental collapse that would come
later in Austin. Starting from childhood, my ego had built up all
these defense mechanisms to protect me from my mom's abuse,
and my defenses held. All my tricks and tools and schemes of
self-medicating and propping myself up, they kept me going. And
therein lies the irony of what the ego does. It creates this armor to

protect you from abuse, but the armor that protects you from abuse is the very thing that allows you to continue abusing yourself. You keep going and rationalizing your abusive reality more and more, wholly unconscious of the fact that your armor is taking a beating and that eventually, *inevitably*, it's going to crack.

By the time I landed in Austin in 2017, I was ready to crack. All of my traumas had started playing themselves out day after day. I was becoming, in the parlance of the industry, "difficult." I had lost faith in the entire system, and in turn I'd lost my faith in nearly everyone in it. There's a reason that actors, often more than those in other artistic disciplines, get pinned with being "difficult." It's because our names and faces are always the ones on the line. If a movie succeeds, we're probably given too much of the credit, but when a movie sucks, we're the first ones people blame. But filmmaking is an extremely collaborative medium. What you see on the screen is the result of the work of hundreds, sometimes thousands, of people, everyone from the set designers to the score composers.

And of all of those people, despite all the credit and blame we're assigned, actors by and large, have very little power over the finished product. The writers, directors, and producers control most of what you say and do. The director and editor make all their cuts, and then, the executives have the final say on what the movie will ultimately be. They have total control over what parts of your performance they want the public to see, and in the wrong hands that can be a career killer. An astute critic or viewer will watch a film and recognize what's the fault of the actor and what's not, but for the average moviegoer, the movie's success or failure is often inseparably attached to the faces that carry you through the story. Any time you make a film or a TV show, you carry a disproportionate amount of the liability for the finished product, but you have practically zero agency or power or control over how that product is ultimately made, other than just showing up and playing your individual role as best you can. For a class of people who are prone to anxiety and problems of self-image to begin with, it's practically designed to engineer a mental breakdown. Add to that the modern pressure of social media, where everyone is judging you and giving you instant feedback on everything you do 24/7, and it's a wonder people can even function.

All of that drama you see played out for public consumption in the tabloids, actors being difficult to work with or having temper tantrums or being divas, those are all manifestations of poor mental health. That person is scared inside. That person is being ripped apart by anxiety and fear. If you help them to be less scared, you will make better movies and everyone will be happier and wiser, not to mention wealthier, because you've made a better movie. But that's not how Hollywood normally operates. It *normally* just milks people for as long as it can and then casts them aside when they're deemed no longer milky enough.

From film to TV to music, the entertainment industry has given us countless examples of immensely talented people who are crippled by poor mental health and who have nobody around them capable or caring enough to shepherd them through the darkness. Yes, you have some agents and managers who try their best, but by and large nobody wants to upset the gravy train. Everybody's happy to keep making money as long as they can still get the monkey to dance. But then once the monkey starts pulling on its rope and refusing to clang its cymbals, then all of a sudden it's like, "Wow, this is a difficult monkey. Isn't it strange that the monkey's throwing shit on the walls after we locked it in a cage and made it dance for fifteen years? But hey, fuck that monkey. Let's go get the hot, young monkey who doesn't know any better."

By 2017, closing in on thirty-seven-years old, I was no longer the hot, young monkey. Having failed in marriage and failed to fix my family or start a new family of my own, the only scrap of self-worth I had left was my career as an actor—or, more specifically, what the grown-ups and decision-makers in Hollywood thought of me as an actor. That was the last piece of the emotional scaffolding holding me up, and it was starting to buckle and fold.

My brief forays outside of TV into motion pictures had yielded me roles in *Big Momma's House 2* , *Thor: The Dark World*, and *Alvin and the Chipmunks: The Squeakquel*, but that was as far as I'd gone. I was becoming this guy who only did sequels, which made me always feel like the runner-up.

My whole career, even with *Chuck*, I thought I was failing because nothing I did ever put me into the next echelon where I was with all the cool kids doing all the cool kid movies and being a part of those conversations. I always felt like I was on the outside looking in, and that wrecked me on a regular basis. I always felt like I wasn't doing something right or I wasn't good enough, and when *Chuck* ended that feeling only multiplied.

The closest thing I had to real success in movies was voicing Flynn Rider in *Tangled*, Disney's take on the Rapunzel fable. It was such an incredible experience and I'm so proud of it, and I think Disney absolutely crushed it. I still meet people all the time who saw and loved the movie, and that's everything for me. But voice-over work isn't accorded the same kind of respect as live action, so it did nothing to move me up to that next echelon.

One of the few developments that pulled me out of my funk, at least temporarily, was getting a call from James Gunn, who was directing the new *Guardians of the Galaxy* film for Marvel. He wanted me to come in and audition for the lead role of Star-Lord. I went in and auditioned. They liked me. Then I got a callback. I got a screen test. This was the actual *lead* in the next big Marvel franchise. I felt like I was *soooo* close. I even started to let myself think, *Oh my God, this might actually happen* . . .

But it didn't happen. Chris Pratt, who was everyone's first choice but who'd been saying he wasn't sure he wanted to do it, finally agreed to do it, and that was that. In the moment, it sucked, obviously, because I had wanted it so much, not fully realizing the reasons why I felt I *needed* it. The psychological ramifications were only beginning, and over the course of the next few years, losing out on that part really started to wreck me.

Chris is a great guy and is super talented, and he deserves every bit of success he's achieved, but for me, in that moment, it was soul crushing seeing his face plastered all over the world. His handsome mug was on every newsstand, every airport kiosk, one after another after another. It was this constant reminder: *You blew it, Zac. You're not good enough. You could have done it. It was so close, but you fucked it up. You just fucked it up.* Chris was off on this incredible trajectory, and I wasn't. At the time, it felt like one of those *Sliding Doors* moments, where you see how your whole life could have changed in an instant and gone a completely different and amazing direction. It was such a bitter pill to swallow.

Of course, that's how it felt at the time. In hindsight, I know that I wasn't ready for the responsibilities that would have come with that blessing. In the emotionally fragile state I was in, if I'd shot to the A-list like Chris had with *Guardians*, I might have crashed and burned in an even more grisly way than I eventually did. In hindsight, I know God was telling me that I needed to prepare myself for His blessings before He could give them to me. But boy, it didn't feel that way at the time. At the time, it felt like nearly all the grown-ups and parents in the industry were united in a chorus of disapproval, telling me I was pathetic and worthless. The only offers I was getting were for more network television shows, which, given my experience with network television, was the last thing I wanted to do.

> The only healthy comparison you can make is with your own self: to be a little stronger, wiser, and healthier than you were the day before.

There was only one place where my career had an actual pulse. While I'd been shooting *Heroes Reborn* up in Toronto I'd hosted this game show for Syfy called *Geeks Who Drink*. It was basically a televised version of the trivia night they hold down at your local bar or pub, a fun but admittedly lower-brow take on *Jeopardy!* That led to a relationship with the folks over at Syfy, and that led to a lot of other cool possibilities, like more game shows or maybe a late-night talk show for their network.

I was deeply ambivalent about it. I was sure if I went down that road, if I became a "TV personality," that would be the end of me as an actor. Goodbye, blockbuster movies. So long, prestige television. I had a hard time coming to terms with the idea, to be honest. Had I built my whole career just to . . . host game shows? But on the other hand, I thought, when I managed to take my own hang-ups out of it, I still felt like my purpose in life was to entertain. And people like game shows. They bring a lot of joy to people, and if that's how God wanted me to bring joy to people, then maybe that was the best thing for me after all. Either way, I desperately needed it to happen because my ego had hung my whole sense of self-worth on my career, at that moment it seemed like Syfy was the last, best, and only chance I had to stay afloat.

I was praying and praying, trying to figure out what God wanted me to do, and part of me deep down felt that God wanted me to get out of Hollywood. Leaving the inhumanity of LA had been a vision in the back of my mind ever since I first started working in the business, when I looked at Hollywood as a whole and thought, *This is broken. There has to be a better way.* That's when I started thinking more about the dream that would become my move to Texas. With digital cameras and the internet and smartphones and social media, all the technology exists to build a studio where people not only work, but also live and play—an intentional community of performers and artists free to do what God intended them to do: entertain, bring joy, and make incredible art. For twenty years, this idea had been percolating in my mind, and the more I grew disillusioned with Hollywood, the more consideration I gave it.

I got it into my head that I was never going to be happy if I stayed in LA. I needed to go and try to make my new United

Artists–style studio dream a reality, because I'd be kicking myself for the rest of my life if I didn't at least try. I was at the point where I realized it was now or never, time to piss or get off the pot. I didn't have anything left to lose. Having researched a number of locations, I prayed and prayed over it and ultimately decided that Austin was where God was telling me to be.

I flew down with a couple of buddies who were business associates at the time. We drove around the outskirts of town, looking at big parcels of land and scouting it all out. Then, about thirty minutes east from downtown, I found it: the Promised Land. "This is it," I said. "I can feel it in my gut. I've gotta go. I've gotta do this." I flew back to LA, sold my house in record time, pulled the rip cord, and jumped, putting most of my stuff in storage and packing the few things I thought I'd need into a U-Haul that I hooked to the back of my truck. Then I drove for two days straight to Texas.

I still believe that getting out of LA and moving to Texas was absolutely the right decision to make, but with hindsight I can say that I probably didn't make it in the right way. In my mind, I was going to fix everything with this one grand gesture, but that is not how something as complex as the human machine gets fixed. I was going to pack up and leave all my problems behind. But when your problems are inside your head and your heart, you always end up taking them with you. Shocker. You can't run away from yourself, as the saying goes. But I tried. I didn't know how sad and broken I really was, and I'd got it in my mind that all I needed was to make a clean break from LA and go create this new world—a thing that would give me the self-worth I was no longer getting from Hollywood. But in the process, I pushed away all of the people who cared about me, and as I sped

> Our ego is an incredible survival tool, but it also holds on to old, incorrect thinking as a bad side effect. Let it go, and we can be healed through a renewing of our minds.

east on I-10 as fast as my truck could go, the darkness I thought I could escape was following right behind me, its shadow looming like a storm cloud high above, ready to swallow me up at any moment. I showed up in Texas with no girlfriend, no family, no friends, determined to do whatever I needed to do to make this new dream a reality. I quit smoking, I quit drinking, and then I lost my mind.

One afternoon, only a few weeks after I arrived, my agent called: the people at Syfy had decided not to move forward with our deal. That was it. I was done. In that moment, the armor that had been protecting me my whole life finally cracked. Since the day I'd discovered acting, I'd been able to survive all manner of abuse and heartache because of the validation and purpose I found in this one thing. Now I'd lost that one thing. I had nothing protecting me anymore, nothing holding me up, and I collapsed. The next thing I knew I was in a small village in the Philippines, sobbing uncontrollably in the throes of a complete mental breakdown.

Not getting to host a game show on the Syfy network was the tiniest of defeats. It was nothing compared to the psychic wound of losing out on the *Guardians of the Galaxy* role or having my marriage fall apart. But it was precisely the fact that it was so insignificant that made it feel so enormous. Even this little, meaningless thing couldn't go right for me. I had invested every ounce of my self-worth in my identity as an entertainer, and now even the thing that I didn't want didn't want me.

I had lost everything, ruined everything. I was a worthless human being. Chris Pratt's happy face was still staring out at me from every magazine cover in the universe, and all I could do was shuffle around Austin like a zombie, thinking about all the wouldas, couldas, and shouldas of the things in life that had passed me by. I didn't know how to love myself, and didn't know how to stop beating the absolute shit out of myself. Luckily, through the grace of God, and help from family and friends, I managed to stumble

my way to Connecticut where I fell through the door of a therapist's office and said, "I don't know who I am. I need to know who
I am and how I got here, and I need to make sure that doesn't
happen again because I don't want to die, but I don't understand
why I should keep living."

# ELEVEN

# Learn to Forgive

It's absolutely necessary to build healthy boundaries with people who've hurt and abused you in life, but boundaries are only one part of it. You can build walls to keep out everyone who's ever hurt you, but you'll still be dying alone inside your own castle if you're not doing the work, *your* work, to get healed.

. . .

As Christians, we always frame Jesus's teachings in philosophical and theological terms, but if you read those teachings a slightly different way, the message of forgiveness is really a super-intuitive understanding of human psychology that was way ahead of its time. Among the many concepts I think Jesus understood better and sooner than anyone else was forgiveness. We all want forgiveness for our sins and our faults. But the only way to forgive yourself is to accept that you were programmed that way, that you didn't have a choice in your parents or how you came up as a child and that's not your fault. But guess what? In order to apply that logic to yourself, you now have to apply that logic to everyone else in the world. The only way to achieve forgiveness for our own sins is to learn how to forgive others for theirs—including our parents.

As has been said many times in many ways, refusing to forgive someone is like drinking poison and hoping that the other person will die. Forgiveness is not only, or even really, about the other person. Forgiveness is coming to the end of your ego and radically accepting that the pain caused by this person isn't personal. It's pain that they're passing on because it was passed on to them. It's generational trauma. It's unhealed hearts and minds damaging other hearts and minds. This is why it's so important to radically accept and radically love yourself and others, at every turn. Finding the way to a place of forgiveness is difficult for anyone. For me, nowhere has it been more difficult than in my relationship with my father.

*As someone who grew up in the Christian faith, I've read my Bible a good bit, and I feel like so much of what Jesus was talking about were ideas that have been ratified and validated within modern psychology.*

There's a powerful scene in the movie *Good Will Hunting*, the emotional climax of the film, where Matt Damon's Will Hunting character and Robin Williams's therapist character both acknowledge the abuse they suffered from alcoholic fathers growing up. All through the film, Will has been putting up his tough-guy act, relying on a lifetime's worth of defense mechanisms to avoid reckoning with his terrible childhood and all the bad, self-destructive choices he's made in the years since, choices that have hurt the very people in his life who are trying to help him. Then, over the course of this one scene, his tough-guy act starts to fall apart as Robin Williams looks him in the eye and then hugs him and says to him, over and over again, "It's not your fault. It's not your fault. It's not your fault."

The reason we're so afraid to confront the problems of our past is because we're ashamed of them. We're ashamed of what we feel. We're ashamed of the bad choices we've made. We're ashamed because we believe those bad choices were our fault—that those mistakes and those feelings of worthlessness are who we are. But they're not. By and large, the trauma and the bad programming that led us to make those mistakes has less to do with us and almost entirely to do with the way that we were raised. We look at the truly damaged people in society, the people who commit awful crimes or hurt other people in unimaginable ways, and we say that they're evil and there's no good in them and our answer is always to punish them and shame them more, which simply has the opposite effect of stopping the madness. Instead of seeing the abused child in them, and helping that child to heal, we dehumanize them, severing from them any amount of empathy or grace, and in turn amplify their propensity to abuse even more.

I don't believe that those people are evil. They may commit evil acts, but they are humans. They're children of God. They're damaged. They're the ones who need to be hugged tight and told, "It's not your fault. It's not your fault. It's not your fault." But of course, it's not that simple, which is one of the tricky things we as a society have yet to figure out. It's said that if we admit that damaged people are not at fault for who they are then we've absolved them and the wrongs they've done are no longer their responsibility. But that's not the case. Both can be true at the same time: it may not be your fault, but it's still your responsibility. When it comes to the way we talk about these issues, we need to reach a point where we understand that explaining someone's behavior isn't the same as excusing it. If you have pain and bad programming and feelings of worthlessness inside you, that is not your fault. But when your pain has caused you to transgress and hurt other people, accepting and dealing with the consequences of your choices is still your responsibility. And that struggle, the difficulty of reconciling those two ideas, is to this day at the root of all of the issues I have with my father.

Just as I was packing up to leave for Connecticut, my dad flew down to Austin with my sister Sarah and some other family friends to celebrate my thirty-seventh birthday and hold me together until I could get into treatment. Late one night he and I were in my living room, sitting on opposite ends of the couch, and I was doing my best to ease him into the conversation I'd tried to have with him on several occasions before. Once I found myself standing in the wreckage of my own failed marriage, I tried to talk to him about everything I was going through and all the ways he hadn't been there for me and how much that had fucked me up. But trying to get him to open up was like pulling teeth. Even with his own son sitting there, crying as hard as I've ever cried about anything in my life, at the last gasp of my ego and self, in so much pain that I wanted to die, he still couldn't do it. Instead, all I got from him was a begrudging, "Sorry. You wanna hear me say 'Sorry'? Okay. I'm sorry!" He did not know how to do any more than that. He didn't have the emotional capacity to go to those depths, nor the emotional vocabulary to say what needed to be said.

And that's not his fault.

My dad was born in 1946 to Alton and Alice Pugh in St. Paul, Minnesota, the second of four kids. When he was young they left the Twin Cities and settled in Amo, Indiana, population around 450, a town so small it's tough to spot on a map. Grandpa Alton was a World War II veteran. The dude was a beast, a man's man, a hero who'd fought in the Pacific and come home with a Purple Heart and shrapnel in his leg. After the war Grandpa Alton helped start the volunteer fire department in Amo, and was so involved in the community that the town renamed the old firehouse/post office "The Alton Pugh Town Center." Just before he passed away in 2001, for his service Grandpa Alton was awarded the title of Sagamore of the Wabash, which is the funny name of the highest honor bestowed by the State of Indiana, something they give to astronauts and politicians and famous actors.

> When I was six years old my dad left me in the care of an abusive, emotionally unstable mother. It took me thirty years to understand that his leaving wasn't his fault. I'm still waiting for him to accept that it is his responsibility.

All his accolades aside, what Grandpa Alton wanted in life was a son to play ball with. Instead he got my dad. Darrell Alton Pugh was not the superathletic, let's-go-be-volunteer-firefighters kind of kid. He was more the sensitive, nerdy, artistic kind of guy, like me. Grandma Alice was very religious, loved church hymns, and taught piano to all of the kids in the area. She had all of her kids singing like the von Trapps all the time. That was more my dad's speed.

My dad didn't do great in school either. He wasn't dumb; it just wasn't for him. He's a simple guy with simple desires, simple needs; he never wants for much, doesn't own much. After a semester of college and a short stint at the phone company, he ended up enlisting in the Air Force right as the Vietnam War was getting into full swing. He spent most of the war stationed in Tokyo, and when it was finally his turn to get deployed to Vietnam, it turned out God had other plans. This other soldier he knew was running some kind of black-market operation smuggling cigarettes and booze and all manner of contraband in and out of Saigon. Having been sent back to Tokyo, he needed to get back to Vietnam to keep his operation going. He asked if he could take my dad's place and my dad, like any sane person, said, "You betcha!"

So while Grandpa Alton spent WWII charging the beaches at Okinawa, my dad spent all of Vietnam hundreds of miles away from the jungle, playing in a rock cover band doing Beatles and Stones hits for evenings at the officers' club. After a postwar stint in Germany, he ended up in Los Angeles for his job, and he was singing in the worship band at church when one day this thin hippie chick with long, wavy brown hair and a big smile walked up to him and said, out of the blue, "God told me I'm supposed to marry you."

So he did.

To look at it in hindsight, if there were ever two people in the history of the world who should never have gotten married, it was my mom and my dad, with my mom and my stepdad coming in as a close second. But at the same time, it makes perfect sense that my parents did get married, because my dad, as Carl Jung would put it, was simply trying to heal the trauma bond he'd endured as a child. In my father's case, that meant marrying a woman *like* his mom to try to heal his relationship *with* his mom.

I didn't grow up with Grandpa Alton and Grandma Alice; they were in Indiana and we were in California, and my mom was a difficult person to deal with, so we would rarely see them. But apparently, like Grandma Pat, Grandma Alice was quite the ball-buster. She'd had a hard life. She grew up on a farm in the Depression, no electricity, only an outhouse for a bathroom, that sort of thing. Her father was an alcoholic and he was gone a lot of the time, leaving her and her siblings and mother to take care of the entire farm. As I've come to learn from my dad's siblings, all Grandma Alice wanted in life was to move to the big city, have a career, and do something adventurous. She never wanted to be married and never really wanted to have kids, but those were the days when that was what was expected of women. So she married a man she didn't really wanna marry, and had four kids she didn't really wanna have. She wound up fairly miserable and hardened because of it, and she took it out on everyone around her. She wasn't physically abusive like Grandma Pat, as far as I know. But she was domineering and controlling. I believe that my dad, being the quiet, sensitive type, never stood a chance.

Instead of learning how to assert himself, my dad learned how to please and appease the larger personalities around him. So when this charming and charismatic California cyclone known as Susy Hoctor blew into his life one day at church and told him God said they were supposed to get married, he was powerless to resist. *This is God's will*, he thought. *It must be God's will.* He just went along with it.

The fact that they met at church, and that my mother presented their meeting as divine providence, was important. If someone walked up to you at a coffee shop and said, "God wants us to get married," you'd look at them like they were a crazy person. But within the religious culture of the time—this hippie-dippie, woo-woo, superspiritual Christianity that had permeated Southern

California and elsewhere—the same pick-up line made perfect sense, especially to someone like my father. My father is very much a follower of Christianity—an adherent in every sense of the word. Prior to the pandemic, he'd never miss church. In fact, he'd go multiple times a week. He'd still sing in the worship band and teach at Sunday school here and there. Now he will drive around with no radio on, or sit in his apartment with no TV on. You ask him what he's doing, and he'll say, "Just waitin' on God. Just sittin' here, waitin' on the Lord." It's deeply ingrained in him to just be with God and wait around for what God has to say. So the fact that he met this beautiful, charming hippie girl in a hippie church played a lot into my dad's thinking.

I think that's one of the hardest parts of my relationship with my dad, our different approaches to faith. We share some elements in our beliefs, and I appreciate his faith, but I think he hides behind it. He'll sometimes use it as a shield, as an excuse. When my mom and dad finally got divorced, he didn't have it in him to fight her anymore. He was cooked. She'd chewed him up and spit him out so much that he didn't have it in him to co-parent with her or even fight her for custody. Then came the moves— ours to Seattle and his to Charlotte—and that pulled us permanently apart. But my dad has always used his faith to gloss over that rupture. He told me many times growing up that he agonized over it and prayed over it, but that he always came to the same conclusion.

"Son," he'd tell me, "I was so worried and I was praying and calling out to God, and the Lord said, 'Darrell, don't worry. They're my kids. I've got 'em.' And I knew you kids were going to be fine."

For a long time, I used to think, "Wow, that's amazing. How cool that God told you that. And look at us, here we are. God did take care of us. We're alive. We're okay."

Except we weren't okay. We weren't okay by a longshot. Because what he did was leave us in the hands of someone who was emotionally and mentally unbalanced, and we suffered the consequences of that and are still suffering the consequences of that now. Our dad could have been a shield, the first line of defense, but he wasn't.

My mom would always wield that fact as a weapon whenever she was angry at him. "Your dad didn't *fight* for you," she'd say. "Your dad didn't *want* you." As a kid I always defended him. "But you're the one who moved us to Seattle," I'd shoot back. "What was he supposed to do, keep following us around?" But now, as I've gotten older and watched my sisters and friends have kids of their own, I've realized, "Well, yeah. That is what the fuck you're supposed to do. They're your kids. They're your responsibility." But in his brokenness and unhealed trauma, my dad had genuinely allowed himself to believe that God had absolved him of that responsibility.

I know that my dad is a good man. I know that he means well. I know that he loves me and my sisters. Occasionally, especially in my teenage years, there were times when I needed help talking through something heavy. That's when, to his credit, he was a good dad. I'd be going through some heavy shit that I could never talk to my mom about because she was so unstable and she might blow up. The pain would build up inside me to the point where my dad could hear it in my voice. He'd ask me what was wrong and I could confide in him about whatever it was, something that I had done wrong or something I'd screwed up that I hated myself for, maybe something between my mom and Gary and their chaos. No matter what it was, my dad never got angry. I could have said, "Dad, I killed someone," and he would only say, "Son, I'm disappointed in you. I know you can do better than that, but I love you, and so does God." On those rare occasions, a few times a year, he could be a real shoulder to cry on and a real voice of compassion and wisdom and encouragement and direction.

My father genuinely cares about people too. He's always been a devout servant in trying to do good in the world. He has always been there for other people's kids, teaching Sunday school and helping out with church picnics and BBQs. Everyone in all the churches he's attended in his life will tell you nothing but the most wonderful things about him. And I'm glad for that. I'm glad that God has been able to use him in other people's lives, but at the same time I think all of that has also been a refuge and an escape for him. It's important to serve your community, obviously, but it's also a less messy way of being a good person. Helping to teach kids who you don't have to take home at the end of the day is noble, but it's far less complicated than taking care of your own.

My dad lived in Charlotte for twenty-five years, and in all that time we never got to visit him there. He never said, "I'd love for you kids to come out here for once." So we never did. It was always just two weeks in the summer on the West Coast, which continued even as I became an adult. All through the years I was doing *Less Than Perfect* and *Chuck*, my dad would come out and stay with me. When he did, he'd visit me on set every day. He'd walk around and everybody knew him and he'd get high fives and he was every-body's pal. He got to be "Mr. Levi"—even though his name is ac-tually "Mr. Pugh"—and I got to have my dad. For a long time, I felt like, "Hey, this is great! I've got my pop!" Except I didn't, really. There was never any acknowledgment of the past, of the pain we shared, and certainly no attempt to fix any of it. It was all very surface-y, like two weeks of swappin' howdies, except in person. Emotionally speaking, he might as well have been back on the other side of the country.

When my dad finally retired at seventy, Shekinah and I were living in LA and Sarah was up in Ventura, so we reached out to him. "C'mon, Pop," we said. "Come on out and retire in LA." So he did. He moved out and got a place in North Hollywood right near me and Shekinah. He even started going back to the same church where he met my mom. Having him around full-time, I made an effort to connect with him on some kind of deeper level, but quickly I found that it wasn't going to happen. I tried getting him to open up about his childhood and relationship with his parents. That didn't work. "It was fine," he'd say. "We got on fine." Which I know from talking to his siblings was simply not true, as they painted a much different picture.

I feel like my dad, in many ways, is still a teenage boy. His parents never taught him to have the confidence or maturity we all need to handle big emotional challenges in life, so the trials of marriage and fatherhood, followed by the trials of co-parenting in a divorce, were simply too much for him. I know my father loves me. But it's not his love that's in question. It's his ability to recognize how much collateral damage was done because of the decisions that he and my mom made, particularly when it came to us kids. That has never been resolved. My dad's inability to handle that without completely shutting down, that's where the breakdown comes. Whenever the subject comes up, whatever script starts running through his mind, he closes down so fast.

And I understand why. I do. Deep down, he's probably terrified. I don't think his psyche can handle it. My dad has felt so much shame in his life. All of the traumas that he endured rendered him incapable of truly standing up and fighting for his own children. But he's afraid to go back and reckon with that because he's afraid it will only bring on more shame. Because that's how we wrongly deal with so many things in our society. When people admit wrongdoing, when they admit they have fallen short, they're rarely forgiven. Too often they're shamed and humiliated. I didn't want to shame and humiliate my dad. Just the opposite. I wanted the healing that lay on the other side of acknowledgment.

As I've gotten to know my dad, it's become very evident to me that his relationships with his parents stunted his growth in significant ways. I can look at his decision to leave and, in spite of my pain, I do understand it. I think it was his survival instinct. I think he felt like he was going to be destroyed by my mother. He didn't have the emotional tools or weapons to fight back against her, so he retreated. I understand that, and I can even forgive that, but I've had a hard time relating to him without an acknowledgment of the pain that his choice caused.

I don't like to speak in ultimatums if I can help it, but after my dad and I failed to have any kind of breakthrough in Austin, as I was leaving for Connecticut, I came close to giving him one. "I'm gonna go do this therapy," I said, "but if we're going to fix our relationship, if we're going to even have a relationship, then we have got to go to therapy together."

He deflected as usual. "Ah, son. I'm seventy-two years old. I'm fine, I'm fine. I don't need all that."

But I needed it, which was something he still wasn't acknowledging. Once I arrived in Connecticut, my relationship with my dad was one of the subjects I was wrestling with the most. What I found, somewhat to my own surprise, was that despite all of my mom's abusive behavior it was easier for me to forgive and find closure with her than with my dad. Part of that was simply that he's still alive and she's passed away; since there's no longer any way for her to accept responsibility, there's no point in getting angry about it. It simply is what it is.

With my dad, I didn't know what to do about the fact that he wasn't stepping up and being the father that I needed or wanted him to be. I was willing to absolve him and tell him I know that it wasn't his fault, but I still wanted him to acknowledge that it was his responsibility and that it had a huge effect on me and my sisters, which he still wouldn't do. And I didn't know how to have a relationship with him if he wasn't willing to do that.

I remember sitting in my psychiatrist's office one day telling him precisely that. "I don't know if I can ever have a relationship with my dad," I said. "Not until he's willing to go to therapy and reckon with all of this."

"Okay," the psychiatrist said. "But what if he never does?"

"Well, then . . . I don't know," I said.

"So let me understand. You're saying you're going to give your dad this ultimatum that he can't be in your life unless he goes to therapy with you, right?"

"Yeah," I said. "That's the whole point. If he wants to have a relationship with me, then he has to go and do this. That's what I need."

"Then your own happiness is still being held hostage by your father, by his being willing or unwilling to go and do this work that you think he needs to go do. If you're waiting for your father to go and do this, then your happiness is going to hinge on something that may or may not ever happen, and so you're potentially never going to be happy—and you might end up losing your father in the bargain."

> I think we need to have a big rethink on what's really important in life. In this world. For all of our futures. And in the meantime, give yourself and others a break.

Up to that moment, I was so upset that losing my father was a consequence I was willing to accept; I was not above cutting people out of my life who I felt were not healthy for me, at least temporarily. But my therapist forced me to wrap my head around the other side of that: what it means to be unable to forgive someone.

Jesus's concept of forgiveness was radical in its time, and I don't think we fully grapple with that fact even to this day. We've glossed over it in such weird ways. We treat forgiveness like it's a traffic fine. The person says, "I'm sorry," and you say, "I forgive you," and that's that. But forgiveness is much deeper and more three-dimensional. Forgiveness is genuinely being done with something. Forgiveness is finding resolution and closure. Ultimately, forgiveness is radical acceptance. It is radical love. It's understanding whatever someone did to you was because of their brokenness, not because of you and not because they are a "bad person." They had bad programming, and that led them to cheat on you, hit you, yell at you, whatever. "Forgive them, Lord, for they know not what they do." It's not a random platitude plucked from the Bible. It's a profound insight into the ways in which generational trauma shapes who we are and how we treat other people, even in ways we do not understand. If Jesus could say that about the Romans who crucified him, who are we to deny that forgiveness to the trespasses others commit against us?

To this day my relationship with my dad isn't what I want it to be. He still maintains in his own heart that he didn't do anything wrong, that God is good and God had a plan, and look how it all turned out with my sisters married with nice families and my being this successful actor and it's all okay. Even if I wanted to get a better father out of him now, I don't think I could. Our relationship has always been pretty surface-level, and it remains that way. It's sad and it sucks and it hurts, but that's life. I know I can't change my dad and I can't fault him either, because I know what he's gone through in his life. I don't feel animosity toward him either. And I haven't made any ultimatums of "You either go and do this therapy or you're not in my life anymore." I see that scared little boy in him, afraid to confront the past, so I've learned not to press it.

I came away from Connecticut with a renewed vision for my relationship with my father. I would radically love him for exactly who he is. If our relationship never got deeper, or stronger, that would be okay—and it is okay. Even if my relationship with my dad isn't what I wished it would be, I've grown to accept that it is the best relationship that it can be. My dad understands that I love him, and I understand that he loves me.

# TWELVE

# *Love Yourself*

If there is any point in this life, it is to love. If you are acting as a conduit of light and love, if that is your only purpose in this world, then you are doing your job—and you are doing it efficiently and at the highest level if you've done it for yourself first. Self-love is putting on your oxygen mask before helping anybody else. When you struggle with loving yourself, then you really struggle with allowing someone else to love you because you don't think you're deserving of it. You don't even know that you're doing that, but you are. So love yourself and go use what you have to be a conduit of love and light and life, and know that if you do, when you are finally extinguished and your time here is through, you will have done your part in this snap of a finger that is your lifespan on this miracle of a fucking planet.

* * *

Of the myriad issues I have had in life, my biggest problem was my unresolved pain and trauma caused by my relationship, or lack of relationship, with my mother. Don't get me wrong, having an absentee father and a highly traumatizing stepfather fucked me up plenty and have absolutely derailed my life in ways that had nothing to do with my mom. Moreover, despite the many accounts of her abuse that I detail in this book, my mother also brought a tremendous amount of good and love into my life. Into others' lives. Into this world.

I believe that my mother tried to love me, and very much did love me, with the understanding and tools available to her at any given time. But she never learned to fully love properly, because she was never fully loved properly, and with that never learned how to fully and properly love herself. That lack of self-love is what I think spawned her narcissistic tendencies. We tend to throw around the word "narcissist" a lot nowadays, so I don't write about it lightly. But I'm also of the mind that we all struggle with bouts of narcissism. The things to ask yourself are just how deep the struggle is and how negatively it is affecting your life and the lives around you. For my mom, her inability to love herself left a massive hole that she didn't know how to fill without making things about herself. Her narcissism was her ego trying to keep her alive. And since she never learned how to love herself, that meant I never learned either.

> Find a quiet place. Sit down comfortably. Close your eyes. Put your hand over your heart. Slowly breathe in and out through your nose. And as you breathe, repeat these words to yourself either audibly or not: "I am loved. I am worthy of that love. I am exactly where I am meant to be."

Before I went to Connecticut, I didn't know that. I didn't know that I didn't love myself. I didn't even understand the concept of self-love. I thought I did. I think a lot of people think they do, but I don't think most people actually do. If you love yourself, you don't speak ill of yourself. You don't chastise yourself. You don't hate on yourself. You don't speak down to yourself. I did all of that, ad nauseam, without thinking twice about it.

Because I didn't love myself, over the course of my life, time and again I've attracted a number of surrogate moms, older women who've recognized me for who and where I was and tried in various ways to protect me, love me, and encourage me. They were essentially moms who weren't my mom, women who felt compelled to stand in the gap for me and comfort me and pray for me.

Unsurprisingly, on my first morning in Connecticut, I immediately fell into a similar pattern with my companion for that day, Beth. I showed up for breakfast that morning and she made me bacon and eggs, which is pretty much the most "mom" thing a person can do. As we got to know each other, not only did I learn that she was the wife of the pastor of the church I'd chosen to attend while I was out there, she also told me that she'd been given my first name a week and a half before I arrived, so she'd already been praying for me daily. It was such an incredibly meaningful gesture of kindness at a moment when I couldn't have felt more unlovable. This woman was incredibly empathetic with what I was struggling with. In fact, she was quite possibly the most empathetic person I'd ever met—the definition of the word. I could feel her feeling my pain, but she was able to do it in a way that never derailed her the way my empathy often derailed me.

Yes, it was her job, but she cared. You can always tell when you're dealing with someone if they care about their work or if they're just punching a clock. There's a marked difference, and Beth was definitely the former. She had a purity about her, a purity of essence. I would almost say childlike, not in a sense of naivete but of joie de vivre. And as pure and wholesome as she was, there was never a feeling as if she had not lived life and experienced pain, loss, and doubt. She had done all of that yet remained this sunny, delightful presence in spite of it. With Beth, I felt right away that she got me, that she felt me. Often when you're struggling with something, you feel your pain is so unique that there's nobody you can talk to about it because nobody will understand it. I never felt that way with Beth. I never felt judged by her. I never felt a lack of understanding from her.

There were five or so different companions who would rotate through on a daily basis. All of them were amazing and full of love and empathy. But with Beth there seemed to be this deeper connection. I ended up having her assigned to me maybe three to four times a week, and the more we talked, the more we discovered these odd parallels between our lives. Beth was nothing like my mother, and her marriage was nothing like my mom's marriage to my dad or stepdad; she and her husband loved each other. But Beth had three kids: two daughters, who were the oldest and youngest, and a boy in the middle, just like Sarah, Shekinah, and me. Like me, her son had also struggled with mental health issues.

It's the sort of thing that people who don't believe in God would chalk up to a random string of coincidences. But for those who do believe in God, you'd say that maybe those things were precisely what they were supposed to be in that time and that place for two strangers to meet and find a connection with each other.

I've always tended to see meaning where others see coincidence. I just have. I've always had a deep faith. Starting when I was a kid, even as young as six or so, I understood faith. I could wrap my little head around the concept that there was a God and that God loved me. I'm never going to say that I know exactly who or what God is, because I don't think that any of us can or will ever understand that, but I've always felt the Creator's presence and love in my life. Or at least I did, right up until I wound up in Connecticut.

I grew up in a very spiritual home, but because my father left us, it was not necessarily a very religious one. While my father's faith ran deep and gave his life the structure and ritual he took comfort in, my mother's faith—surprise, surprise—was the exact opposite. My mom took us to church almost zero times. Occasionally, if we were visiting friends in another place and they had a church that they liked, we might go pop in, but it was rare. We did go to this church camp in the summertime, but that was a day care more than anything else. I'd say we probably went to Catholic Mass with Grandma Pat more than we ever went to church with my mom.

My mom, as we know, had massive problems with authority. Part of that was due to her personality, and part of that was the era she and my father had grown up in. America saw a lot of upheaval and change in the 1960s, and Christianity was no different. The old hierarchical top-down models of the Catholic church and the mainline Protestant faiths, all of that was being called into question. People like my mom were rebelling against that, giving rise to what people call the hippie-Jesus movement or the Jesus Freak movement. As with other hippie endeavors, it was throwing off the expectations of what society was supposed to be and figuring out who you were and who God was for real. It was all about "expanding your mind," but with Jesus instead of LSD, although some sects probably dabbled in both. Which is how you end up with my parents getting married the way they did, my dad with long hair and a big Grizzly Adams beard in a brown leisure suit and my mom in a white summer dress with a flower crown in her hair.

But where my dad eventually settled into a more traditional expression of faith, my mom did not. There was no structure, no discipline to her spiritual life. I think she didn't like going to church, in part, because she thought she was smarter and more in tune with God than the pastors. And hey, she probably even was sometimes. My mom struggled with authority partly because of ego, but also actual experience. The church where my parents met and thrived for years started to devolve into a crazy cult after a while, which caused them to get outta there real quick. Couple that with the long list of numerous corrupt church leaders throughout human history, and it's no wonder my mom had her trust issues with organized religion. So my mom's walk with God mainly consisted of her getting together with her like-minded friends, talking about politics and spirituality. She'd have dinner parties with a bunch of people and they'd talk all night, praying and reading the Bible and feeling the Holy Spirit and speaking in tongues—all that fun, spirit-filled stuff.

Growing up in that household, and feeling God as instinctively as I did, for a long time I simply took faith as a given: God exists and the Bible is His Word. Then I turned eighteen and started to ask myself the age-old question: "Do I really believe in this stuff, or do I believe in it because my parents believe in it?" I wanted my faith, to be *my* faith. That's when I decided to start pursuing God and understanding God on my own.

My entire life I've gone back and forth between something like my father's approach to religion and a path closer to my mom's. Sometimes I'll find a congregation I feel called to and attend services regularly and faithfully for months or even years. Other times I'll find myself gathering a few friends for Bible study and home church, as I did for many years in Los Angeles, and I'll root my faith and my community there. Either way, church—meaning the actual people who are gathering—has always been a powerful and wonderful part of my life. So when I found out that first morning that Beth's husband was the pastor of the church I had randomly picked out, my connection to her felt even more like it was meant to be.

My first Sunday in Connecticut was a rainy day. I woke up, and Beth picked me up and drove us over for the service. I liked Beth's husband. I didn't have the opportunity to get to know him terribly well, but he seemed like a kind, gentle man. I could understand why he and his wife loved each other and had such a healthy relationship because, seemingly, they were cut from the same cloth. They were people who loved people.

It was a nice service. I sat in the back, and Beth sat one row in front of me. I can't recall what the sermon was, but I do remember that it was good. When the worship music started playing to wrap us up, on a better day, I would have been the guy standing up, hands in the air, praising God. I've always preferred a more cathartic, charismatic service, filled with the Spirit. I've always felt like if we're going to church then we should be celebrating that we're alive and we have each other and God loves us. Which I never really felt when Grandma Pat took us to Catholic Mass. I didn't find God at Mass. I felt liturgy. I felt ritual. But I didn't feel like it was communing with God. The same thing was always true at the more staid, conservative mainline Protestant churches as well. It works for a lot of people, and that's cool for them, but it was never my cup of tea. I've never felt that that's what church was meant to be. I go to church hoping to learn and grow but also sing and clap and feel God's spirit in me.

But not that day. I was so wrecked and so low that I couldn't even muster it. I even started crying during the praise and worship music. Not like crazy wailing, but I just sat there, softly weeping. Everyone around me, clapping and singing, could feel the Spirit, but I felt nothing. I couldn't feel God. His love had left me, completely. Had I reached the point where I didn't believe there was a God anymore? I had been through ups and downs with faith before. I had been through seasons of doubt, as we all have. But never like this. At the end of the service, Beth's husband invited anyone who wanted to come up to the front to be prayed over. So I went up and got prayed over by a bunch of lovely people in front of the church. It didn't help. It wasn't enough to fight off all the doubts and darkness. I still felt spiritually dead inside.

So, seemingly abandoned by God, my last bit of faith was now vested in all these expensive doctors and therapists I'd hired to save me. "They're the best of the best," I thought. "If they can't help me, I don't know what I'm going to do." By the second week I was starting to feel better. I was learning so much about the human mind and mechanism, why I was stuck repeating so many of the unhealthy patterns and behaviors that had crippled me my whole life. Just like the old cross-section illustrations in my favorite book *The Way Things Work*, my therapists had cracked open my cranium and shown me—to the extent that medical science knows—where the gears and pulleys were and how the whole contraption had broken down.

It felt, haltingly, like progress. Then, at the beginning of my third week, I started plunging down again, fast. Suddenly I was leaving my appointments feeling worse than when I had gone in. I felt like I was back in Austin again, circling the drain. As illuminating as all my sessions were, nothing had actually improved. In fact, all my baby steps of progress were, in many ways, only making me feel worse. I kept having these breakthroughs with my therapists that gave me new insight into my marriage, into the generational passing of trauma, into the nature of true forgiveness, and everything else. But all this new knowledge and insight did nothing to drive out the sadness and self-loathing that consumed me. It was like lighting a match and having this fleeting moment of hope, only to see the tiny light snuffed out and the darkness return.

One of the primary values of therapy, that the counselor is a disinterested third party, is also one of its primary drawbacks. Many of my sessions felt impersonal and clinical. I'd be sitting in these therapists' offices, curled up in a ball in my chair, bawling my eyes out, snot and tears running all over the place, and the most they would do would be to gesture to where I could get myself a tissue when what I needed was a fucking hug. I needed someone to grab me and swaddle me and hold me through my shaking and my crying and tell me it was going to be okay. But therapists don't do that. They can't do that. Which I totally get. I understand the need for a doctor to maintain a professional distance and not get emotionally involved with patients. It's for your benefit and theirs. But that was what I needed: someone to be emotionally involved with me, someone to hold me and love me and support me because, try as she might, my mother was too traumatized herself to do it properly, and I never learned to do it myself. So I would leave these appointments feeling even more disillusioned than before. If this last-ditch, pull-out-all-the-stops therapy wasn't helping me, then nothing would ever help me, which is about the most hopeless feeling there is.

But I'd come out of these appointments feeling terrible and there, sitting in the car waiting for me, would be Beth, this surrogate mother praying for me and showing me unconditional love and support. The companions at this place had a strange role. On the one hand, their job was to be there for you and support you in whatever way they could. But it was supposed to be a logistical role, providing transportation and breakfast and so forth. It was expressly outside their job description to provide any kind of therapy or guidance or counseling of any kind. Which, again, I understood. In any medical environment, there has to be a clear distinction between laypeople and licensed professionals. Beth was allowed to be a shoulder to cry on, and no more. But she ended up being so much more. She would sense the pain and frustration in me walking out of these appointments, and she'd take me for a drive somewhere to help me clear my head and heart. Sometimes we'd grab a coffee and drive down to the state beach and go for a walk to get me out of my own head for a bit. Most times we'd drive down to the waterfront and park and I would be crying and screaming at the top of my lungs, which is something I had been doing a lot since Austin, just being on my knees screaming and crying out to God for help, crying out in anger and frustration.

While I was breaking down, often Beth would be tearing up—not weeping, but there were some real raw, tender moments where I could feel her feeling me. I could feel her empathy. She would offer a lot of deep spiritual reminders, telling me that God loves me and is there for me and that she was there for me and, although this was a difficult season, it was preparing me for what was to come. Nothing groundbreaking or revolutionary, just basic truths. Things that might seem trite if you saw them on a motivational poster, but coming out of the mouth of somebody like Beth, no matter how ridiculous they might sound because of how jaded you might feel, you could hear the truth in them because she's so full of love and light.

Honestly, it was less about what she said and far more about her presence and how she allowed for that space for me to kick and scream and cry and yell. She would sit with me and pray with me and I didn't have to say anything. I would say that, at that point, I felt that I'd lost my faith completely. I didn't know if I believed there was a God anymore. But at no point did Beth ever say, "You're wrong. God exists." At no point did she try to cheer me up by saying, "That's not true." She just prayed for me and encouraged me and reminded me that I was okay, that I was safe, and that I was loved. She didn't preach God to me. She was just there as a godly presence in my life. It felt like I finally had a healthy mom at thirty-seven. I finally had a warm, loving woman to do all these little things to make me feel safe, and feeling safe made me realize I had no idea how unsafe I'd felt my entire life. I'd never even registered what that felt like because it was just normal, and here was this incredible woman whose actions and words were showing me how abnormal it really was.

Then one morning, about halfway through the third week, I went to my regular appointment with my psychiatrist. I actually woke up that morning feeling optimistic, but by the end of the session I was teetering on the brink again. I was so angry, so despondent. I had no idea what was going on with me or if there was ever going to be any kind of diagnosis or a course of treatment I could follow. I shuffled out, thinking, *What's the point? This isn't getting me anywhere.*

Beth picked me up, and I immediately started breaking down in the car. She drove me out to this point on the water and parked, and I sat there in the passenger seat, tears streaming down my face, screaming as loud as I could. My voice was gone, shot. She didn't say a word. Literally, not one word. But I knew that in her silence she was praying for me, quietly resting her hand on my back, giving me reassurance that I was going to be okay. She allowed me to fall apart and be in my brokenness without judgment.

Eventually, my anger subsided, and we sat there for I don't know how long. I slowly pulled myself back together, she started the car, and we drove off. As we were heading back to the house, Beth turned to me. "Just so you know," she said, "what I'm doing, praying for you, I technically shouldn't be doing it. They don't want any of the companions to do anything that could potentially interfere with the programming that you're receiving while you're here."

"I won't tell anyone," I said. "Just please don't stop praying for me. I don't care about their stupid rules. I need it. I need it in my life. You're helping me fight to stay alive."

We drove on for a beat longer, then she turned to me and said, "But also know that I would gladly lose my job for you."

The moment she said that, I lost it. I would never have asked her to lose her job, or put her at risk of losing her job, but the fact that she was willing to do so, that she would be so selfless as to make that kind of a sacrifice for me, was almost too hard to believe. To go from how I'd been living my whole life, my mom staring me down and saying, "I'd be happier today if you were dead," to this woman telling me she was willing to lose her job to pray for and love me, it was be-

> Don't beat yourself up for not being there yet. Pat yourself on the back because you're on your way.

yond comprehension. It was such a simple gesture but such a profound one. Now, between the clinical help from my battery of specialists, coupled with Beth being an incredible conduit of God's love and grace, I truly began to turn a corner. I felt this incredible catharsis, a flood and rush of emotions and warmth inside me. I felt like for thirty-seven years I'd been drowning, fighting and kicking to reach the surface, and in that moment, I finally broke through and filled my lungs for the first time. I felt grace with myself. I felt like I could forgive myself. I felt like I could love myself. And the more I felt I could forgive and love myself, the more I felt I could forgive and love my mom, my dad, my stepdad, and everyone else in my life.

Time with Beth was like time with the healthiest version of my mom, which was unfortunately missing all too often in my life. In reality, she was in many ways a complete stranger. But it was the fact of her being such a stranger that made her love and prayers and sacrifice that much more powerful. Like an angel, she was an instrument of God who helped pray and love me back to life.

Beth's actions played a major role in what ultimately saved me in Connecticut. Without her, I don't know if that would have been a successful journey. Which is not to say that the therapists and professionals weren't good at their jobs. They were. What they gave me was vital and necessary to my healing process. But because of the clinical and professional barriers, they couldn't show me love, which was a massive part of what I needed. To be loved. To be shown love. To be guided into the understanding that I am worthy of loving myself. Beth was tuned into God and understood that. Then she made herself available to be the instrument that God used to help me see and feel that more clearly.

I think a lot of people go and get treatment, and the reason their treatment doesn't ultimately hold is because they leave there learning a lot and knowing a lot but still feeling like a piece of shit. They don't have a person to hold them and say, "You're loved. You're worthy of love." That was certainly the case for me. My deepest ailments, my inability to love myself, my inability to recognize my own self-worth, could only be fixed with love, by another human being loving me in order to show me the way to loving myself.

Despite everything I had learned up to that point, my depression and pain and agony had persisted because of the one thing I still did not understand: Knowing how to fix a machine is not enough. Ultimately, you have to believe that the machine *deserves* to be fixed. That you are worthy of the healing you seek.

# THIRTEEN

# *Keep Going*

It's not a sprint; it's a marathon.

. . .

By the time I left Connecticut, I thought I was good. I had gone through this therapy, done this deep dive, and was earnestly on the road to finally loving myself. I felt like that was God telling me I was back on me feet. I knew I wasn't out of the woods entirely, but I felt like I had a compass and a map and I knew where I was going. I felt like I could look forward to some smooth sailing, at least for a little while. Maybe some future trauma would come along and fuck with me, but as far as the past was concerned, I thought I was good to go.

I was wrong.

Maintaining your mental health is a lifelong process. It's not a one-and-done. It's not "I got sick. I took antibiotics. Now it's gone and I don't have to worry about it anymore." Or, to compare it to caring for your teeth, if you don't brush and floss and stay vigilant, you're going to continue to have problems. Even if you go and get a root canal, if you don't start practicing proper care and maintenance of your teeth, you're just gonna keep needing more root canals.

I think part of the reason I was in denial about the never-ending aspect of coping with mental health was that, at the time, it felt like such a downer. It was depressing to think that I'd never put it be-hind me, that I would always be wrestling with these demons. I don't think that way anymore. Learning to deal with our trauma and learning how to love ourselves is simply the business of life. It is part of what it means to be a life-form on this little blue dot. It is neither good nor bad—it simply is.

More than that, however, seeing mental health as a never-ending struggle actually helps you. Once you see this as a journey with peaks and valleys, once you understand that the good times won't necessarily last forever, that gives you the perspective to finally understand that the bad times won't last forever either. There is always a dawn that follows the darkness.

The morning after my breakthrough with Beth, I woke up to an email from one of my agents. Since everyone on my team knew not to bother me unless it was absolutely necessary, I was curious what was so urgent that this email had to be sent. So I clicked it open. "Hey, Zac," it said. "So, we know you're on a retreat and we don't mean to bug you, but there's another role in *Shazam!* they'd like you to read for. It's a supporting role. The scene is attached. If you want to do it, you can put yourself on tape. If not, no wor-ries. There's no pressure. We're just throwing this out there."

Reading it, my initial reaction was to laugh, to be honest. The irony that Hollywood wanted to have me back to potentially smack me around even more while I'm literally still in therapy working out the initial beatings—it's pretty funny when you think about it. Twisted, but funny. And it wasn't my agency's fault. I hadn't told them the extent of how bad things had gotten, only that I needed some time away. Plus I was only just coming to understand the role that work had played in my poor mental health myself, so I couldn't expect them to know. Still, it wasn't an email I was ready to receive. I was still so unsure about my state of mind, about every-thing. I wrote back and said, "Hey, I need some time to process this. When does this need to be submitted by?

"No problem," they wrote back. "End of day Friday would be great."

For the next two days, I went about my regular appointments, mulling over what I should do. For so long I'd had so much of my self-worth wrapped up in what Hollywood thought of me, in thinking I was a failure because I hadn't achieved everything I thought I was supposed to achieve. And I'd *barely* reached a point where I could acknowledge that that wasn't true, that I hadn't wasted my life, that I was where I was, and that was okay. But then I remembered that in life God is always using us for a greater purpose, for other people's lives and the benefit of the world. We don't get to dictate how that's going to go, and maybe this email, this opportunity, was God reminding me that we always have to give our best to whatever is right in front of us.

So as Friday rolled around, all of that was sinking in, and I had the teeniest little pep in my step from the breakthrough I'd had with Beth. And the material was funny too. I liked it. It had a bit of back-and-forth dialogue at the beginning, but it was basically a monologue, so I could read it on camera by myself. Eventually, I decided to do it. I told myself that it wouldn't affect me if they didn't like me or if it didn't go anywhere, because I wasn't going to let my self-esteem get wrapped up in the answer. So that afternoon, I finished up my workout at the gym, headed back to my room, and, still wearing my sweaty workout clothes, I took my phone and propped it up precariously on the dresser, using two books to pin it at the right angle. Then I hit *record* and did the scene. I did the first take and liked it. Then I started to do a second take, and I kind of flubbed it halfway through, so I stopped. Then I thought, "Well, I liked the first one, so whatever, I'll send that one." I attached the file to an email and sent it off into the ether.

That was around 5:30 p.m. Connecticut time, which means it was around 2:30 in the afternoon in LA. I didn't think I'd hear anything back until the middle of the next week, at the earliest. Then, about an hour later, my phone started blowing up. It was my agent.

"Hey," he said. "So, uh . . . everybody saw your tape, and not only did they love your read, but they think that you could be their Shazam."

"Wait, *what?*" I said, completely in shock. "That's crazy. I thought they cast it a month ago."

"Nope," he said. "That didn't go through. They've been camera-testing different people, but they haven't nailed the role down yet, and they think you could be their guy. They want to know if you can put yourself on tape for the part. It's three scenes."

Unlike the monologue I'd done, all of them required a signifi-cant scene partner to act opposite, and I didn't have anybody I could read with because I was in this house in the middle of a tiny New England town excavating thirty-seven years of emotional and psychological trauma. I couldn't exactly go to my psychiatrist and say, "Hey, would you mind running some scenes with me?"

"Well," I replied, "I'm in the middle of deep therapy in Con-necticut, and I don't have anybody to run these lines with."

"Can you fly in?"

He wanted me to *leave?* Leaving meant missing out on my last week of wrap-up sessions with my doctors. "No," I said. "No can do."

He told me to stand by, and after some back-and-forth with the film's producers, it was decided that I would audition via Skype the following Monday for the director, David F. Sandberg.

Monday afternoon David called, and we chatted a bit. I told him I was sorry I couldn't be there in person because I was away at this healing retreat, and he was cool with it. Then I took my iPad and he took his iPad and he hit *record* on his end and, with his casting director reading the lines through the screen to me in this house in Connecticut, we ran through the scenes. We did it twice, maybe three times. It was pretty quick and easy. I said, "Cool, thank you very much. Have a good day," shut down my iPad, and went back to my journey of healing. I felt good about it, to be honest. I didn't want to go getting my hopes up, but in the back of my mind I kept thinking, *I wonder how this is going to play out.*

I didn't have to wonder long. Maybe a half-hour later, my agent was blowing me up again.

"Okay, so here's the deal," he said. "You gotta come to LA. Warner Brothers says they want to fly you in for a proper camera test, not you on an iPad. They need that. It's between you and one other guy. If you don't come in, they're going to give it to him. If you do come in, the tide is shifting in your favor, and there's a strong possibility you'll get this job."

At that point, my head practically exploded. I started pacing around my room. My mind was racing. *What the* fuck *is going on here?* Part of what had put me in this place, after all, on top of my mom and everything else, was that I'd been so needy for approval that I'd allowed myself to suffer so much getting chewed up in the Hollywood machine. I'd taken my entire sense of self-worth and handed it over to some people who didn't really value me as a human being. Now, it felt like Hollywood was saying, "Hey, leave the place you're at—the place we helped put you—and come back. We have this shiny new thing for you. It's your wildest dreams come true. You'll be a *superhero*! Finally!" I felt like Michael Corleone from *The Godfather Part III*: "Just when I thought I was *out*, they pull me back *in*!"

The whole thing felt strange. I was obviously skeptical. All these alarm bells were going off. Was this God testing me? Was this the darkness tricking me? Because I knew it had to be something. This wasn't normal. Either this call was the culmination of the work I'd been doing in this place, God opening a door for me because I was ready to handle it, or it was a lure of the flesh trying to take me away from finishing the work and getting in a truly healthy frame of mind. I'd only completed three weeks of therapy, and I still had six days left. And while by that point I was actually feeling much better and stronger, how was I to know how ready and healed I was? I didn't even know if I was healthy enough to go back to my regular life, let alone go and carry a major Hollywood superhero movie with thousands of people and hundreds of millions of dollars depending on me. As the saying goes, with great power comes great responsibility, and I was still struggling with being responsible for myself.

I went downstairs and found Beth. Given how much I needed her on this journey, I have no doubt God was responsible for putting her on duty that afternoon. I pulled her aside, laid out the whole situation for her, and explained my dilemma. I went through all the reasons why I shouldn't do it, but then there were also all the reasons why I felt like I should. In some ways, it just felt right. I'd always dreamed of playing a role like Tom Hanks in *Big*, being a kid who magically becomes a grown-up, and here was that same story only with superpowers, which was such a fun idea to play with. On top of that, the story of Shazam has a Biblical connection as well—albeit a subtle, yet still profound, connection. It's a story set in a world of gods and demigods, and the main enemy is the Seven Deadly Sins. I'd be playing a superhero whose name is an acronym that starts with "S"—"S" for Solomon, the wisdom of Solomon. Movies about mutants and radioactive spiders are cool, but this was about a godly/godlike man fighting literal sin incarnate. I mean, c'mon!

Then there was the character of Billy Batson himself: an orphan, abandoned and rejected by his own mother. I wasn't an actual orphan, but I might as well have been in some ways. I kind of had parents growing up, but I kind of didn't. And I certainly didn't have any parents after I was twenty-one. I looked at this character and saw so much of myself on the page, this kid who wants to find acceptance and family. I suppose you can find correlations in anything if you're looking hard enough, but I felt so many connections to the story and the character that I had to believe it was more than mere coincidence.

"Beth," I said, "I honestly don't know what to do."

"Well," she said, "let's pray about it. Maybe we'll hear something or feel something."

So we did. We sat down on the living room sofa and prayed. After a few moments, we both looked at each other, and we both agreed: This wasn't some trick. It was the fruit of my coming to Connecticut and doing the work that I'd been doing. And the reason I knew that was true was because when I prayed I felt . . . nothing. I didn't feel the crippling anxiety or the jittery nerves that I'd felt, you know, for most of my life. But I also didn't feel giddy about it. I wasn't getting that sugar rush of approval I'd become addicted to, the thing that kept me going every time I performed or landed a gig. What I felt was the absence of those things, a lack of that anxiety and neediness and fear. I felt at peace. Which felt *incredible*. I knew that I could go to LA and audition for the job and, if I got it, that would be cool. And if I didn't, that'd be cool too. It wouldn't be the end of me. My sense of self-worth wouldn't hinge on this.

> We will be known by our fruits. And if one's fruits aren't those of love, joy, peace, patience, kindness, goodness, faithfulness, gentleness, and self-control, then there's a good chance they are the false prophets we've all been warned of.

Even as my faith has evolved over the years, one thing I have always held on to is the power of prayer and its ability to bring peace. And if prayer has real power behind it, Beth was absolute proof of that power. Faith the size of a mustard seed can move a mountain; I think Jesus talked about ideas like that for a reason. Ultimately, I'm not sure any of us can say who God is in all their facets and capacities. But it's people like Beth who genuinely believe in the power of prayer, and her faith was bigger than a mustard seed, I can attest to that. It is said that wherever two or more are gathered in God's name, God is there. And on that day, with Beth and I praying together as two, I found the peace I'd been searching for. I'd started this journey with Beth, and I ended this journey with Beth. She helped pray me back to life, and now she was praying me into the next part of my life. It felt genuinely, perfectly, poetic.

I went straight to my room, called the administrator, and explained the situation, saying that I thought I was in a good place, but I needed her to confer with my therapists to vouch for that fact, because I didn't want to make that call on my own. She did, and a few hours later she emailed me to tell me everyone was confident that I was good to go. I went up to my room and started packing.

The next morning, I came downstairs to find Beth. I took her aside, and we shared a brief moment. We exchanged a few tears and some very honest words. "Zac," she said, "it's been a privilege to be God's vessel of a momma's love for you." "You literally helped save my life," I told her, "and you will always be *in* my life, whether you like it or not." We both shared a laugh, said our goodbyes, and I was driven to the airport where I caught the first connecting flight to take me out to Los Angeles.

After a long day of airports and taxis, I checked into my hotel in Hollywood and got a good night's sleep. The next morning, a production assistant arrived to take me to the Warner Brothers lot in Burbank, rolling up in this little white Honda Civic. I remember how small it was because it was not designed for a person of my size; not many cars are, I suppose. I folded myself into the front seat next to him, and off we went, chatting along the way. He was this eager, earnest, affable kid—he honestly reminded me of myself when I was starting in the business. It was sweet to look over and be reminded of the way I used to be and to think about all the miles I'd traveled and everything I'd been through in the years since, all of which had led me to this moment.

Once we arrived at Warner Brothers, we went up to the New Line Cinema offices, and I was escorted into the room where David and his casting team were waiting. Before we ran the scenes, we talked for a bit about the character and the story. The whole time I felt the same peace I'd felt while praying in Connecticut. We ran the scenes a couple of times, with David stopping to give me direction here and there between the takes. The whole meeting took, I don't know, maybe half an hour, start to finish. Finally, he said, "Okay, I think I got what I need."

"Cool," I said. "Thanks very much."

Then I walked out, folded myself back into this guy's little Civic, rode back to the hotel, and that was that.

That afternoon I checked out and called my buddy Eric to see if I could stay at his place for a couple of days while I waited for the news. He said I could crash on his futon, which wasn't even a futon but one of those miniature foam couches that kind of pulls out into something like a mattress on the ground. But I tell you what, even on that thing, I didn't toss and turn one bit. Everything was cool.

The next morning, I got up and went to the gym to work out. I was on the bench press in the middle of a set when my phone rang. It was David.

"Hey," he said, "it's David Sandberg, and I'm calling to let you know that you're my Shazam."

And even then, in that moment, I was at peace. I didn't rocket to the moon or feel some sense of validation filling an empty chasm inside me. It just felt right. I told David how grateful and excited I was. Then I said, "Well, thank you very much, sir. I'm going to get back to the bench press now, as it seems I'll need to be doing this a lot. We'll talk soon."

Moving forward from that day, I actually let myself think, *Okay, marathon finished. Finish line reached. I'm okay.* And for the next couple of years, my mental health was pretty solid. Prior to Austin and Connecticut, I had a therapist in LA I saw during my divorce. I went back to him and I was talking to him every other week or so, and he helped a lot. I still had some rough moments here and there, for sure, but for the most part I was okay.

I wrapped up filming *Shazam!* and then flew to New York to do *The Marvelous Mrs. Maisel*, and that felt great because not only was I working with all these incredible people, I was finally getting to be a part of an award-winning show that got all the respect I always wished *Chuck* had received.

The only real problem during that time was that I still had all these digestive issues that were (theoretically) somehow linked to whatever I'd picked up in the Philippines. I'm still convinced that problem has been and continues to be a huge factor in my body chemistry being jacked up. It's scary to have some undiagnosable, undiscoverable, very real problem inside of you. The hypochondriac in me was like, *Is this cancer? Am I dying?* It also breeds a great deal of distrust in the whole medical system, making you feel helpless and defeated and alone; I've since learned lot of the issues people have with parasites go hand in hand with anxiety and mental health. Finally my doctors discovered this amoeba in my body and prescribed me medication for that, and once I took it, I felt considerably better and my mind felt considerably better as well.

> Once we share some vulnerable moment about ourselves, it's insane how many people go, "Oh my God, me too!" So I don't ever want to hide and not talk about the struggles that I've had.

Once *Shazam!* came out, I found myself with the biggest media platform I'd ever had. I was flying around the world on press junkets from Beijing to Mexico City, and I told my publicist from the beginning, "Hey, the only reason I'm even here to publicize this movie is because I went and did all that work on myself. So I think it's my responsibility to use this opportunity of promoting the movie to talk about my mental health journey to getting this role, as much as I possibly can. It will be an incredible way to normalize and destigmatize mental health issues in general."

They were receptive to the idea and, in addition to the usual late-night talk shows, I went and talked on a number of podcasts focusing on mental health and wellness and spirituality, shows like *Inside of You with Michael Rosenbaum* and *On Purpose with Jay Shetty*. It was a lovely, groovy experience. The conversations were engaging and inspiring, and even after *Shazam!* had its moment and moved on, those conversations kept going on Twitter and Instagram. People were responding to the messages I was putting out about the need for self-love and self-worth, and among those doing the responding were some folks from the publishing industry who thought my story might make for a compelling book.

I'd been asked about writing a book on previous occasions, and my response was always the same: I'm not famous enough or important enough to merit an autobiography. I haven't even lived enough life to fill all those pages. But HarperCollins, after hearing my Jay Shetty interview, was convinced that I had a book in me specifically about this. Not an autobiography, per se, but a book about my journey to better mental health. I still wasn't sure I'd be able to handle it, but it had felt rewarding to share my stories through podcasts and social media, so I decided to give it a try. I sat down back in Austin and I started working with an editor. We were cranking out pages, and meanwhile my film career was enjoying a nice post-*Shazam!* bounce. I popped down to South Africa to work on *The Mauritanian* with Benedict Cumberbatch for a bit. I had a movie lined up to start filming in Cleveland, and then the *Shazam!* sequel was all lined up to film in Atlanta after that.

And then: Covid-19.

In those first early weeks after the Covid-19 lockdowns started in March 2020, I was—believe it or not—filled with optimism and hope. Not that the pandemic was good or exciting, mind you, but because times of crisis in history have so often worked to bring people together with a sense of community and common purpose: The whole nation rallying together after Pearl Harbor. People climbing in boats to rescue their neighbors during a flood. Like a lot of people, I initially thought the pandemic could be that sort of catalyst. On top of which, my engineer's mind loves problem-solving and finding solutions, and here was one very big problem in need of many different solutions. Hollywood was shut down, meaning all of my friends in Hollywood were unemployed. Somehow the industry was going to have to figure this out, and maybe I could help by getting a bunch of people to quarantine together in this big, open space I have in Austin and we could keep working, helping each other and doing what we love. *This is going to humble us as a species and galvanize us as a nation*, I hoped.

Well, I was wrong. That didn't happen. Instead, the opposite happened. Everything about the response to the pandemic became polarized and politicized almost instantly—it was just another thing for people to fight about on social media. Then, the plans I had to get some work kickstarted down in Austin didn't materialize, on top of which a couple of my friends who were there working with me had to leave. So nothing was moving forward at all. Then George Floyd was killed in Minneapolis, and the whole country blew up in a fit of anxiety and anger and fear, far worse than anything I've witnessed in my lifetime. Because of the way we're all connected to each other now, those tragedies are that much more damaging to everyone's mental and emotional well-being. And with my empath's heart, I couldn't take it.

My breakthrough in Connecticut had been a genuine turnaround. It had pulled me back from the brink and stabilized me when I desperately needed it; I couldn't have shouldered the responsibilities of *Shazam!* if it hadn't. But what was also true, and what I only realized in hindsight, was how much my work was still buoying me, how much I was still relying on external supports to give me those little dopamine hits to tell me I was doing okay and give me feelings of self-worth. The truth is that my life was going well because my life was going well, and the minute it stopped going well, I would spiral back down again. I thought I had been doing everything I could to mitigate the issues I've always struggled with, but I wasn't doing enough, clearly, and I hadn't healed enough not to fall apart.

The pandemic was another perfect storm, the same as my first Austin breakdown, a confluence of events that conspired to obliterate me. It clipped my wings and put me in this freefall.

One thing about working, aside from the little dopamine hits of self-worth it gives you every day, is that you don't have a lot of downtime to sit around and beat yourself up. Under a quarantine, you've got nothing but time to beat yourself up. A lot of people did find a way to use the crisis to find and build a positive purpose. Some people did band together in a positive sense of community, bringing meals and medical supplies to isolated people in need. Others used the enforced isolation and downtime to take on whatever projects they'd never been able to make time for, like painting the house or arranging all their digital photo albums. A healthy person is capable of doing that. They get up every morning and say, "Oh my God, I have all this free time to invest in myself, I'll finally learn how to play guitar. I'll get to work and write that screenplay!" Then, once you do that, you've got the positive feedback loop going. Every day you've got a few more pages of screenplay or you've learned a new chord on the guitar and you feel like you're accomplishing something. I couldn't do any of that. I was back to hating myself, not loving myself enough to want to invest in myself at all. I was waking up in the mornings with major panic attacks. I was utterly depressed, crying and shot through with anxiety and fear for myself and for the world.

Meanwhile, my editor was sending me back pages on the manuscript for this book. By that point, it was practically done. All but finished. Polish up a few sections, clean up a few typos, and it'd be ready to go. Writing a book, unlike acting in a film, is largely a solo affair. It's you and a laptop, and the collaboration that's required between you and your editor happens mostly by phone and email anyway. It might be the most quarantine-friendly creative endeavor there is. When all my other projects dried up, in theory, I could have pivoted all my energies and all my time into this and kept working. But I couldn't bring myself to do it.

During my first Austin breakdown, I couldn't unpack a box of plates and put them in the cabinets for fear that I would screw it up, and if I screwed up my cabinets and my cabinets weren't perfect, then that would mean I was a worthless failure who didn't deserve to live. Which is a typical train of thought for an unhealthy mind. This time, it wasn't a kitchen cabinet that maybe one or two other people might see and judge me for. It was a book that was going to go out into the world and get reviewed on websites and sit on bookstore shelves for everyone to see. If it wasn't perfect, then everyone was going to shit all over it and me, and I'd be even more of a worthless failure who didn't deserve to live. When I opened up the Word file from my editor, I was as paralyzed as I'd been by that box of plates. I couldn't even read past the first page. *Is this even any good? Why is that sentence like that? Should that comma be here or over there? This is* shit. *Why am I even writing this? Why did I think that a worthless fucking failure like me could even write a book in the first place?*

Hoo boy. It was intense. On top of that was the fact that the story I'd told in the book wasn't true anymore. The progress that I'd made in Connecticut was genuine, and the breakthrough I'd had with Beth had led me to a place where I truly felt I understood and had the answer to my problems: I'd been so focused on learning how to fix myself when what I needed to learn was that I had to love myself enough to believe that I deserve to get fixed. Beth's love and prayers did that for me; they helped put me on the road to recovery. Now, either that wasn't true, or it was partially true but still woefully incomplete. It couldn't be the final stage of my journey, because here I was in August 2020, sobbing uncontrollably on my couch in the darkness, right back where I'd been when the story began in August 2017. How was I supposed to write a book helping other people with their mental health journeys when my mental health journey seemed to have taken me around in a fucking circle? In my mind, I'd written an incomplete book, poorly, and I was not in the right headspace or the right heartspace or the right spirit to fix it.

The manuscript file sat there on my laptop for over a month, with me unable to touch it for fear that I'd put a horrible book out into the world that would make everyone think I was an even bigger failure than I already thought I was. At some point I was going to have to call HarperCollins and admit to them what was going on. I was loathe to do that because it would mean I actually *was* a failure, because I had failed to finish the book. The last thing I wanted to do was disappoint anybody by not hitting a deadline and not keeping my professional commitments. I was scared and I was embarrassed. Despite my many struggles in life, all through my various professional endeavors, I was always afraid of disappointing the authority figures on my jobs because if I disappointed people, they would hate me and never want to work with me again.

Eventually, I screwed up some courage, called my editor and my agent, and laid it out for them. "I still want to do it," I said, "but I can't do it right now. I don't know how to write a book about radically loving myself when I don't, currently, radically love myself." Fortunately, they were incredibly gracious, as I hoped that they would be. It was a healthy reminder that, no, not everyone in the world is my mother. Not everyone reacts to disappointing news with whiplash anger and emotional violence. The world is full of people who accept you as less than perfect and understand why you're less than perfect. They agreed to put the book on pause and told me to go take as much time as I needed to put myself back together again.

So that's what I did.

# FOURTEEN

# *Find Grace*

You may feel that no matter how hard you've tried, it's simply not enough. That somehow you have not, and will not, live up to whatever standards have been set to deem us worthy. You may feel that while others deserve these things, you do not. After having gone through my own darkness, and finding light on the other side, I can assure you that you are deserving of kindness. You are deserving of love and patience and forgiveness. Most of all, you are deserving of grace.

. . .

The fact that I stumbled and fell during the pandemic was not, in fact, the problem. I thought it was, but it wasn't. The problem was that I saw it as a problem. The problem was that I felt shame, again. I felt like I'd failed, again. I fell right back into my lifelong pattern of berating and beating the shit out of myself for not being good enough, which was ridiculous. The whole world was suffering from the isolation and dislocation of going through this global crisis. Millions of people were struggling with the same personal and professional issues that I was suffering from, but I couldn't see that. I could only see my own pathetic, worthless self, screwing everything up like I always did.

The road to better mental health is a long and difficult one. You will stumble and fall. You will slip up in a thousand little ways, daily. You will fall backward into old, destructive patterns, again and again and again. And if you treat every one of those setbacks as a personal failure, you will never make it. The only way forward is to get back up, dust yourself off, and move forward again. The only way to do that is to accept yourself as less than perfect. And the only way to do that is to have grace.

By the fall of 2020, I was spent, exhausted, depressed, and generally wrung out. Not only was I feeling like I was failing at life again, but during my international press tour for *Shazam!* I had contracted yet another parasitic infection that, again, no doctor seemed able to properly diagnose or treat. Depression, compounded by a seemingly undiagnosable, unfixable problem inside your body is a recipe for disaster. A friend of mine said, "Maybe you need to go see some spiritual healers or try Eastern medicine." I had tried seemingly everything at that point, and I was willing to do just about anything, so I gave it a shot. I flew to LA and had these different appointments with a kinesiologist and a breath-work healer and an organ-massage healer. But I kept struggling and breaking down every morning. None of it seemed to be working, and as each new thing failed, I felt more and more like a failure and continued the downward spiral.

> One of the pillars of self-love that can be done anytime, all the time, is self-patience. It's particularly helpful when you *are* busy.

It was the same with work. For all those early months of the pandemic, I kept trying to get a bunch of people together down in Austin to work on something and it kept on not coming together. I could have looked at the situation like, "Hey, we're in the middle of a global pandemic and I can't figure out how to mount a film production and *that's okay* because nobody else has figured it out either. It's not a reflection on my value as a human being." But I couldn't do that. Instead, all I could say to myself was, "I'm failing at this and I'm failing my friends and I'm failing God and I'm failing myself because I'm nothing but a useless fucking failure."

I wouldn't give myself a break, and I never have. It's one of my single greatest battles, never having grace with myself, never having the patience to let myself fall down and get up and try again, never having the perspective to say it's okay for something to not be perfect the first time around, or the second, or the third. Any time things aren't happening correctly and quickly, any time I don't do everything as perfect as I think I should, I'm consumed by debilitating feelings of shame and self-loathing.

That October, some of the studios started to put Covid-19 safety practices in place in order to resume production. All the projects I was supposed to be working on remained in limbo, which meant I was now available for other roles I hadn't been able to take. I was cast in a film about the life of NFL quarterback Kurt Warner that was about to start shooting up in Oklahoma City. I was beyond relieved to get back to work, but at the same time I was still hurting inside, wracked with feelings of anxiety and self-doubt.

Then, right after I landed in Oklahoma City, I was talking to different friends of mine about my situation and three of them, right in a row, all gave me the exact same advice: they asked if I had tried antidepressants. I gave them all my usual explanations and rationalizations for why I was wary of them. I'd only tried them briefly and to little or no effect when I arrived in Connecticut, and I had quickly weaned myself off them when they didn't seem to be doing anything. Then *Shazam!* had come along, and at that point I felt so good I didn't see the need to even revisit the idea of them.

Part of the reason for it was the way I was raised, with my mother being into organic food and alternative and homeopathic medicine way before anyone else. I'm happy to have medical interventions when they're necessary and justified, like with my digestive issues, but I don't like putting anything in my body that isn't naturally supposed to be there; I don't even like taking aspirin if it's not absolutely necessary.

The other reason is that when you grow up a Christian, you're told that God has all the answers. He is capable of healing any and every part of your body. Most Christians don't apply this thinking to physical maladies, although Christian Scientists are known to forego medical procedures out of the deference to and dependence on the healing powers of God. But many Christians, certainly the ones I've been around and grew up with, treat mental health issues as a malady of the spirit, not a physiological ailment. After a while, you become conditioned to believe that all of these mental and emotional issues have one solution, and that is seeking God—pray it away, as the saying goes.

But I also know that the deeper reason I'm so ambivalent about taking meds is because of my failure to have grace with myself, my constant need to beat myself up for any kind of personal shortcoming, real or imagined. To admit that I need medication would be to admit that I'm incapable of figuring this out and getting through it on my own without the help of some pill, which would mean, once again, that I've failed. And if I'm a failure, then I'm worthless and pathetic and stupid and all the other put-downs I say to myself unconsciously, all the time. Accepting medication would also mean accepting that I might need it forever, which would mean that I'd never get past this and I'd be stuck feeling like a failure for the rest of my life, at which point why even go on living?

I know a lot of that stems from my own pride and fear and bad programming and flawed logic, but the other big piece of it stems from society's longstanding judgments about people who need those kinds of medications. Although it has changed for the better in recent years, for far too long we labeled people taking medication for mental illness in all sorts of negative ways, and I couldn't bear to be slapped with those labels. Still, as I talked to my friends from my rental house in Oklahoma, they all said, "Zac, I understand your hesitation. I had it too. But antidepressants have changed my life for the better, and I think you should try them because they're basically the only thing you haven't tried yet."

Around the same time I was also listening to this podcast called *The Hilarious World of Depression,* which is a fantastic show. They get a lot of comedians or comic actors or writers to come on to talk about their mental health struggles, issues, and journeys. Just hearing those people gave me a lot of courage. I was like, "Holy fuck, I super respect this person, and would love to work with them, and they deal with anxiety and depression and take antidepressants and it's no big deal. Maybe I am beating myself up too much about this. Maybe I do need to cut myself some slack."

So I called up my therapist in LA, the one I'd talked to on and off over the years who had helped me through my divorce. We talked and I gave him all of my reasons for resisting medication up to that point, and he gave me this great analogy as a way of thinking about it. "Imagine you're in a room and it's pitch black," he said, "but you know that there's a light switch right above you and a stool right at your side. The light switch is too high to reach, and in order to turn it on you need to stand on the stool. So, you step up on the stool and hit the switch. Once the light comes on, you can finally see everything around you clearly. That's antidepressants. It's nothing more than a stool. It's the assistance you need to get above the darkness and see clearly. So give yourself the stool right now to do the thing that you need to do in order for you to not require the stool anymore."

> It takes the deepest courage to be our truest self.

To which I said, "But what if I need the stool for the rest of my life?"

To which he honestly replied, "You might. Look at type 1 diabetics. They have to take insulin every day to survive, and no one judges them. No one sees them as failures."

And he was right. It is okay. I can see that now with the benefit of hindsight and experience.

Talking with this therapist also gave me the closest thing I'd ever gotten to what I was looking for in Connecticut: An answer.

A diagnosis. What is my condition? Why is my brain the way that it is? This therapist believed at the time that perhaps my depression may have been brought on by obsessive-compulsive disorder, or OCD.

When people think of OCD, they usually think of what's been popularized in movies: people unlocking and relocking doors or washing their hands five times in a row. I've always had some obsessive tendencies, not so bad that it was ever debilitating or that noticeable to others, although I do remember being a child and actively having to fight some of those urges. I've always had a thing about symmetry and balance. I couldn't have a nightstand on one side of my bed and not the other. My shoes were always tied in perfect mirror image to one another so the laces crossed the same. Little things like that. But the real manifestation of my OCD wasn't about the need for a systematic ordering of specific objects. It was about the need for a systematic ordering of life.

Whenever I find myself at a crossroads, I'm desperate to make the right choice but I'm utterly unable to divine the right choice, and the end result is a kind of analysis paralysis. I'd get stuck in these thought loops and ruminations and I'd sit and spin and spin, unable to decide anything or pick any one option, which then would make me feel like a complete failure, and then from there it'd be a nosedive straight to the bottom, ruminating and regretting everything in my mind all the way down into a deep, deep hole of anxiety and depression.

And so, the thinking goes, because that obsessive-compulsive feedback loop is creating these problems, if you can break the loop, then maybe you can stop the depression. Prozac, which my therapist prescribed, is indicated to do precisely that. Like most antidepressants, Prozac is a selective serotonin reuptake inhibitor, or SSRI. It deals primarily with your body's ability to regulate its serotonin levels.

So I started taking it, introducing it into my system by slowly upping the dosage. The first couple of weeks were okay but it wasn't doing much for me until I upped the dosage a bit, and then it really kicked in. When you start on an antidepressant they tell you the side effects, and part of the problem with antidepressants is that some of the side effects are the very symptoms you're trying to fix. It's like taking diarrhea medication and one of the side effects is shitting your pants. Prozac, it turns out, can cause anxiety, and for the first three weeks I was on it I had greater and more consistent anxiety than at any other time my life. I was back to work, which I was super grateful for because it distracted me, but it was super gnarly.

Having chemically induced anxiety was helpful in a way, because I was able to separate the anxiety from myself. I could say, "Zac, this anxiety is tied to nothing but this medication. You're not actually anxious; your mind and body are reacting to this medication and hijacking your thoughts. You have to breathe and know that this is going to go away." Diving deeper into meditation practices, I was able to take control of my own thoughts and fight against the anxiety, which helped me make it through.

Once the dosage settled in, I felt lighter, not so serious, more capable of going with the flow and letting things go. I wasn't sitting around beating myself up about shit all the time. My ruminating eased up too. Obviously I was still thinking about life and pondering the different outcomes of my actions, but it wasn't as obsessive or as paralyzing as before.

After a few months of dealing with Prozac and its side effects, coupled with learning more and more about hormones like serotonin and dopamine, I started to wonder if there might be a different drug that offered a better pharmaceutical fit. My therapist switched me over to Wellbutrin and phased that in while phasing the Prozac out to see if Wellbutrin had as good of a stabilizing effect without the other side effects that I didn't want to endure. Wellbutrin is a norepinephrine-dopamine reuptake inhibitor, or NDRI, and it has turned out to be a life-changer for me. It has unlocked for me, finally, what I believe may be the key to understanding my condition, at least from a chemical, physiological perspective.

As I mentioned at the beginning of this book, dopamine is the chemical in our bodies that serves as the motivation for virtually everything we do. Serotonin is more of a love drug. It gives you a steady feeling of "things are okay." Dopamine is a reward drug, a little jolt of excitement. Andrew Huberman is a neurobiologist at Stanford who knows an awful lot about dopamine and the like, and listening to him speak on the subject has been a revelation. Apparently, there was a study done with rats where they surgically removed the ability of the rat's brain to create dopamine. Then they put the rat in a cage and put food right next to it. The rat sat and sat and sat and starved to death. It never ate the food, because there was no dopamine reward for doing so. Dopamine deficiency is the reason why some people with depression, like me, get crushed by that feeling that we can't even get out of bed because we can't do anything. That whole sensation of "What's the point?"—that's a dopamine deficiency, because without dopamine our bodies feel that there *is* no point. Humans need that dopamine reward to motivate us to do the basic tasks like eat and clean ourselves.

When I look back, what I see clearly is that all my life I've been addicted to something, anything, to bring me happiness. Whether it was video games, rollerblading, or entertaining people, I was probably addicted to it. I discovered those diversions and I binged on them the same way other people do with drugs and gambling and food. I always needed to go and find and do more to make myself happy in order to get away from the chaos of my home life and my abusive parents and being bullied at school. I had no idea that the whole time I was bingeing on those things, what I was really doing was jamming down as hard as I could on the levers in my brain to create as much dopamine as possible to make me happy. Just like the Enneagram said, I was making myself a glutton for joy and pleasure and happiness in order to avoid pain.

But there's a serious downside to that. Among the scientists who study dopamine and its effects, one consensus is that the pleasure created by dopamine is controlled by a lever in our minds: the pain/pleasure lever. Pain and pleasure, it turns out, are deeply correlated with each other. Our brains light up in almost the exact same way when we experience either of them. Back in the hunter-gatherer days, there wasn't so much going on in the way of "fun." You were hunting, you were gathering, you were making camp, you were building a fire. You were tracking a bear for twenty miles and then having to kill it with your tribesman. These things sucked. Maybe there was a little time at the end of the day to sit in a circle and tell some stories or go off and have sex, but that's about it. A lot of early life was pain and endurance, and what researchers have found is that when you press down hard on the pain side of the lever, once you let up on that, your body steps in to counterbalance the lever. It rewards you with a rush of dopamine to bring your body back into equilibrium, and man, it feels good. It's why some people get addicted to ultramarathons and going to the gym, because the rewards are so intense.

> One of my fears about going to Connecticut was that I was afraid I wasn't going to be me when I left, because a lot of the traits that made me "me" came from my trauma, so how could I possibly still be me if I left those traits behind?

But the flip side is true as well. When you overdose on pleasure, you have to pay the piper on the other side. In trying to self-medicate my trauma, I was overdosing in pleasure. Whether it was hearing the roar of the crowd or a weekend-long party with friends, I was trying so hard to feel good. Then, when these perfect storms would come along, like a relationship ending or being out of work, I would lose my ability to keep pressing on the pleasure side of the lever and it would flip hard the other way, causing me to plunge far deeper into the darkness than any healthy, well-balanced person would. That is the downward spiral of dopamine deficiency.

Once I started taking Wellbutrin it made me, quite literally, into a more "well-balanced" person. It evened my dopamine levels out. Because I was no longer plunging so deep into the pain of dopamine deficiency, I felt less of a need to go out and self-medicate with the gluttony of pushing down on the pleasure side of the lever. We all think that we are in full and constant control of our minds and hearts, but we're not. We think we are, and some of us are very good at it, but our bodies, biochemically, can be hijacked. And if you don't understand that your body can do that, you'll fall into that trap more often than not.

We are so much more capable of being grateful when we're not battling through the anxiety or the depression or the OCD that hijacks our thoughts and emotions. That's where I find myself now with all of this, and what a difference two years makes in my ability to be more present and have more faith in myself and where God's taking me and what the future holds for my relationships with my friends and my family and everything else.

When my sisters and I moved my mom into her new Santa Paula apartment, Shekinah, true to her word, kept going up and checking in and spending time with her. But over the course of the next seven years, my mom grew progressively worse and worse, more mentally unstable and physically unwell. Shekinah would call and say, "Okay, I'm coming up tomorrow to visit." Then, inevitably, my mom would drink herself sick the night before and call back and cancel, or just not open the door when Shekinah arrived. Eventually, she was doing that with everybody.

As the years went by, pretty much everyone in the family had cut off communication with her entirely. The only real contact we had with her were the drunken voicemails she'd leave, always saying the most toxic, most hateful things, like that I was a bad son and a fucking bastard, the same old song. The ones that followed the end of my marriage were especially rough. "You fuckin' *blew* it. Of *course* it's falling apart. You don't know how to be a *man*. Nobody is *ever* going to love you." I already wanted to die, and here was my own mom leaving me these insanely horrible voicemails. It was dark. I always listened to them though. Maybe I shouldn't have, but I thought I needed to know how bad she was getting. The way she was treating herself, we all knew she wasn't going to be long for this world. We just didn't know the end was going to come as fast as it did.

The call came in the early morning of October 8, 2015, two days after my mother's sixty-fifth birthday, less than a week after she'd failed to make it to Shekinah's wedding. It was my Uncle Mike who called. "I hate to be the one to tell you this," he said, having a hard time putting the words together, "but your mom died last night."

It socked me right in the gut. I sat and I cried and cried. I was crying for my mom, and for myself, but I think I was also crying because I knew what was going to hit me as soon as I picked up the phone to call my sisters.

When I was twenty-two years old, I had a buddy, Mike, who died in a car crash. It was so bad that even with a seat belt and an airbag he was killed instantly. That was the first time I had to confront the death of someone I was close to. I was so young, and at that age you feel bulletproof. I had never contemplated my own mortality, how fragile life can be, how you can be in a car having a great time one minute, and the next minute you're gone.

At the funeral, I was crying and looking around, and every time I made eye contact with someone and saw the sadness in their eyes, I saw Mike dying all over again. It wasn't just that Mike had died in my life—he was dying in all our lives. I realized I wasn't just mourning my friend, I was mourning the loss that each person felt because he was now gone. People don't die once. They die a thousand times, over and over again, every time someone who loved them feels that loss. My mother had already died for Uncle Mike and for me, and now she was going to die again the moment I told my sisters.

I texted them first, asking them if they were free to get together so I could share some news in person. I couldn't reach Sarah, but then I got ahold of her husband and he said he'd find her and tell her. Shekinah was living only fifteen minutes away from me in Glendale, and luckily, she was home.

"Hey, what are you up to?" I texted. "Are you at work? How soon can you be at the house?"

"Soon," she replied. "What's up?"

"Just come over. I want to talk to you about some stuff."

Shekinah made it over to my house, and I sat her down and told her. It was one of the hardest things I've ever done in my whole life. And she knew. "I knew that's what you were going to tell me," she said as she collapsed into tears. We sat there together for a while, holding each other and crying and remembering the good times, the times when Mom was healthier and happier. The salad days.

Over the next day or two, the whole extended family started coming together up in Ventura. My sisters, my cousin, and I went over to my mother's apartment to go through her stuff, to sift through the proverbial rubble. I had never been there. Sarah had only been maybe once or twice. Even Shekinah, who'd been my mom's primary caretaker, hadn't been there for quite some time.

We walked in, and it was like a hurricane had hit it. There was so much hoarding of all kinds of random, weird shit. That's when we met the guy who was staying with her, the guy who'd found her. Even to the end, even as her own life was circling the drain, my mother had never given up on taking in strangers and people who were even worse off than she was; I think that was one of the only things keeping her alive, the fact that there was somebody else she could help and provide for. This guy had been homeless in Santa Paula. He was a broken person himself, a lost lamb, and he needed help. She'd met him on the street and had been bringing him food and clothes and was trying to get him on his feet so she decided to let him stay with her. I think he helped her by going out for groceries and booze, because by the end she'd become a complete shut-in. She hadn't left the apartment for several months.

It was sad going through and seeing what had become of her. Even by our high school years, she was already pretty scattered and not particularly clean or organized, but it was nowhere near this. I mean, shit was everywhere, piles of tchotchkes, junk she'd bought on clearance racks. One whole bedroom was nothing but clothes. There were boxes and boxes of baby clothes. Baby clothes for people she didn't know who didn't have babies. Baby clothes for the grandchildren she didn't have from the children she wasn't talking to.

There was also a ton of old vintage clothes of hers that she would never let go of, shit that I even remembered fighting with her about. "Mom, you haven't worn that in ten years. You don't need it. Let it go. Throw it out." The irony being that now so much of that stuff was hip again and she probably could have made a killing with it on eBay. "Hey, is that a cheetah-print leotard from 1987?! Take my money!"

The other bedroom, the master bedroom, was technically her room but she didn't even sleep in it anymore. She'd given it to this guy. She was sleeping on the couch. She basically never left the couch. She was binge-drinking vodka like crazy. She'd drink and then binge on some junk food to get something in her so she could drink some more and then puke and puke and puke. The irony was that as a young woman she'd been so ahead of the curve when it came to organic food and homeopathic medicine, but her mental health was so decrepit and unstable that she'd reached this point where she physically could not take care of herself.

After going through some of her things in the living room and the bedrooms, I finally made myself do the thing I'd been dreading. I walked down the hall to the bathroom where the roommate had found her. He'd woken up around three in the morning to go use the restroom, and when he opened the door he found here there on the floor, hunched over and not responsive, and he called the paramedics. The coroner's report came back saying that she died of complications from pneumonia, a condition that no doubt had been brought on and aggravated by her drinking and not eating well and refusing to go to the doctor.

In the days ahead, there was plenty that needed to be done: all the housekeeping one has to do when somebody dies, calling the funeral home, reaching out to friends and family, and so on. All of that fell to me, and I was happy to do it because I knew my sisters were in worse shape than I was. I wept for my mom, and I wept hard for about three days. Then the tears turned off. I went back into survival mode. I told myself that I'd mourned her and dealt with it and put the pain behind me, and now I was ready to carry on.

We had a big wake for her at a friend's pub in Santa Paula. We had a band play. We had pictures of my mom all over the joint, pictures of her when she was younger and healthier and happier. It was truly a celebration of her life, and it was beautiful and amazing. So many people showed. So many friends and family came out, such a weird and wide variety of people, people from my life, from my sisters' lives. For a woman who spent her whole life burning bridges, it was astonishing and also very telling. Nobody wanted their bridge with my mom to be burned; everyone knew deep down that she wasn't a bad person. She was just seriously ill and no one could convince her to get help. People genuinely did love her. People genuinely enjoyed her friendship when she was in a good place. She was just never able to stay in that good place for very long.

It's sad when people don't think that they're loved, and it takes them dying for everyone to be able to come back together and celebrate them. Knowing how much pain my mother suffered in life, and knowing that she wasn't in pain anymore, allowed me to tell myself that her death wasn't a tragedy. In that sense, I could see it as a kind of gift, and I held on to that thought as a kind of silver lining. But there was no escaping the overwhelming sadness we all felt, because it *was* tragic. It was tragic that such a beautiful, talented, intelligent, charming, dynamic, and vibrant woman ended up destroying herself without ever being able to live the life she could have lived. It was tragic that she died without ever having the opportunity to reconcile with her parents, her siblings, her ex-husbands, or her children. When you know that somebody is going to die, even someone you've had major issues with, you still want to be able to let them know that you do love them before they're gone, and the fact that we didn't get that chance is one of the saddest and hardest things about losing her the way we did.

When I arrived in Connecticut I genuinely thought I'd made my peace with her. I remember thinking I'd forgiven her because I wasn't actively walking around thinking about her, being upset with her, or stewing on the things she had done. There was a homework assignment I got from one of my therapists in Connecticut. It was to write letters to my parents, telling them how I felt so that I could begin to grapple with those feelings and let them go. Writing the letter to my father wasn't easy. With someone who's still alive, it's a challenge to come to a place of total acceptance and forgiveness without attaching a bunch of conditions and demands about how we want them to change. Writing a letter to someone who's passed away is a different challenge entirely, because that door has closed forever. When I wrote to my mother, I got out a piece of paper and I sat there and stared at it. It probably took me ten minutes to start writing. Every time I tried to put pen to paper I would start sobbing uncontrollably. I had so much emotion bottled up inside of me that I didn't even know where to begin. Then, when I finally did, the first page was a diatribe, me ranting on and on, "And then you did *this* to me, and then you did *this* to me . . ." I couldn't stop crying the whole time. Then I flipped the page over, and honestly when I did it was like my perspective and understanding flipped over in that instant as well.

> We can choose love, or we can choose fear. All other things spring forth from that one decision. I choose love. And I will choose to believe that if enough folks finally do, we will all be free. Every last one of us.

"But," I wrote, "the reason you did those things was because you were broken and hurting, because you didn't feel loved by your own mom, and that's so sad." In that moment, my heart broke for my mom. My heart had never really broken for my mom before because of all the pain that she had inflicted on me. In that moment, it finally did. And the floodgates were opened and gushing. I could see the little girl in her who'd been abused. I could acknowledge that what she did to us wasn't her fault, and I finally felt the grace and the empathy to truly forgive her.

In the end, I know that my mom did love me and my sisters. She succeeded in showing us that she loved us in quite a few ways and moments throughout her life. With someone like her, it's easy to only focus on the negative and not remember the good times that were had, in large part because the good times were so long ago and had gradually faded from view. But we should remember them. Because I do believe, ultimately, that my mom, my dad, and my stepdad all loved us in the best way they knew how, with the tools that were given to them by their parents. I think most "bad parents" do love their children; they just don't understand how to do it in a healthy way. We grow up thinking they don't love us. We grow up thinking they don't care because those are the cues we're receiving, not realizing the way they're parenting is merely a reflection of how they were parented, and so the story goes.

I was fortunate, in a sense, that I did get a message from her to tell me that deep down she loved me too. In her apartment, going through all the random clothes and other shit, I stumbled across a box full of news clippings and articles about me and my acting career, which told me that she was proud of me, even if she was too messed up to ever tell me. But I'll never be able to do the same for her, to tell her how much I care. Maybe she knows. I hope she knows. Once we die and rejoin the energy that is God, I don't know that we even care about life in this world anymore, but if we do, if we can know anything from beyond this life, then my mom must know how much I love her, and did love her. But it's still sad to know that she died alone on her bathroom floor thinking that she was not loved, that her own children didn't care about her. That's what broke my heart the most then, and that's what breaks my heart the most now.

. . .

As I write this, I'm working on a new film, and that's always something that buoys and uplifts me. The real test will come when and if work bottoms out again. That's when I'll know for sure how much support the medication really gives me. I'm going to try to get my body to a place where I won't need it anymore, but only time will tell, and I'm not going to judge myself one way or the other, so . . . we'll see what happens.

Just the fact that I can type the words "we'll see what happens" is a massive leap forward for me. Until now, the decision to take or not take medication had been precisely one of those fucked-up OCD feedback loops exacerbating the problem. If there is always a correct choice, is the correct choice for me to take the medication or not take the medication? Of course, as I now understand, there is no correct choice. Not for that. You go and you try to do things in earnest because you're trying to care for yourself. Maybe it works, maybe it doesn't, but in doing that, you're hopefully finding more tools for your tool belt along the way.

The moral of the story is not "Take medication and it will solve your mental health problems." Medication might help you, or it might not. The importance of the medication for me, beyond its actual physiological effects, was the pivotal, seminal turning point it symbolized in my journey. When I left Connecticut, I'd had a genuine breakthrough, believing that I finally was able to love myself enough to want to heal myself. Accepting that I might need medication, that I might need that stool to stand on to escape the darkness, was the moment I was finally able to say that I can still love myself even if I'm never able to fix myself. It was the moment

I was finally able to stop beating myself up for failing to be this perfect version of who I thought I was supposed to be. It was the moment I finally learned to have grace with myself. True grace. God's grace.

I've amassed so many important tools in the past three years— meditation, prayer, the Enneagram, different therapeutic practices, better eating, better exercise—but simply having access to those tools would be meaningless without loving myself enough to use them and having grace with myself, forgiving myself, every time I fall short of where I want to be, which will inevitably happen. That's life. For the longest time I was obsessed with "fixing" my brokenness, when what I needed to do was *heal* it. As it turns out, there's a huge difference between the two. Fixing is a solution, a task with an endpoint. You follow steps one through four and then you're done and you mark it off your checklist. You're coming at yourself from a technical, analytical standpoint. "What's the problem? Let's get at the problem. Let's solve this. Let's do this." And you think that you're loving yourself because you're trying to help yourself, when the reality is you're not being patient or kind to yourself because all you're doing is judging yourself on whether you're fixing the problem or not.

Healing, on the other hand, is a process. It's an ongoing process, and it's never done. From a motivational or an attitudinal standpoint, you come at yourself a lot differently if you're trying to heal than if you're wanting to fix. To the extent that you are applying more grace and more empathy and more love to yourself as you are navigating behavioral patterns in your life, you are healing more than fixing. Healing is acceptance—radical acceptance. It's being patient with yourself and not beating yourself up over unmet expectations, either yours or other people's, and not basing your worth on external validation.

And I never learned to have grace with myself, or patience or forgiveness—because of that glass of water. Because I had parents who struggled to have grace and patience with me, with each other, and even with themselves. The only way I learned how to treat my-self was to be condescending, impatient, harsh, and critical. That was the only way I knew how to talk to myself. And that's not what good parenting is. Good parents help their children to tackle be-havioral issues by being patient and sitting down and telling the child that there is no shame or condemnation in what they've done, and that they love them regardless. All of these things seem so obvious, but they aren't to so many parents. Or, more likely, parents think they're doing them correctly, but they're not.

We always want to look at abusive people and say, "You shouldn't treat people like that. You should know better. You're a bad per-son." But everyone out there, and I mean *everyone*, believes that they're the good guys. Everyone is the hero of their own story. My mom, for sure, thought she should have been awarded a trophy for Mom of the Year. I have no doubt that in all of her yelling and screaming, she thought she was doing the right thing to fix what-ever was "wrong" with her rowdy, rambunctious kids. She didn't know how to sit with us and our issues, because our issues were a reflection of her issues, and that was too much for her to handle.

My mother didn't love herself. She never learned to have grace with herself. Because it's hard. I wake up every morning and those old habits and that bad programming are still there and I start to slip, and I have to remind myself to love myself and have grace with myself. It's a daily practice. But I do it because I know that practicing radical love and radical acceptance are the difference between breaking the cycle of generational trauma and continu-ing it. They are all that stands between the fate that I've avoided and the fate to which my mother succumbed.

• • •

So, where to from here? I think it's important for people to talk about mental illness because it's one of the key ingredients to solv-ing the problem. Silence is one of the major contributing factors to people feeling inescapably stuck in their depression, their anxiety, their stress, their fear, their shame. If you're suffering in silence, you're not going to find a solution for it, because nobody knows. And we are not capable of getting ourselves out of a lot of these issues that we are facing, mentally and emotionally, particularly in today's society, by ourselves. We need help. We need each other. We need community. We need a tribe. We need family.

I'm convinced that all of the issues that we suffer from in this world are rooted in the broken heads and hearts of individuals. If we could go trace all of that down and heal it, we'd be taking care of the planet, we'd be taking care of the animals on the planet, we would be taking care of each other and ourselves. We'd be doing that because we would not be acting out of our unhealed traumas, or allowing ourselves to be led around by our broken egos in a constant state of fearing and fighting, which is ultimately where all our issues lie. But if we can all acknowledge these traumas and seek to heal and free ourselves from them, then perhaps we can start to truly listen to each other, learn from each other, and radically love each other.

That is my prayer.